WHEN GOD SETS THE TABLE

A Faith-Based Guide to the Healing Power of Food

CARRIE K. CYPRIAN

divergent expressions publishing

When God Sets the Table: A Faith-Based Guide to the Healing Power of Food

ISBN: 978-1-7355701-1-2

This book presents the research and ideas of its author. It is not intended to be a substitute for consultation with a professional healthcare practitioner. Consult your healthcare practitioner before starting any diet or supplement regiment. The publisher and author disclaim responsibility for any adverse effects resulting directly or indirectly from information contained in this book.

Printed in the United States of America.

Cover Design by: B.J. Cyprian
Edited by: Lori Fish & Brenda Green

Author's Note

The reason why I wrote this book:

My purpose in writing this book is a little boy named of Aaron. He was born in 1999. When he was four months old he was given to me to take care of because of his health condition. His diagnosis was "Beckwith Wiedemann Syndrome." He was born prematurely after only 23 months gestation weighing two and a half pounds. Aaron stayed in the hospital for four months when he achieved the weight of five pounds. He was being fed through his stomach by G-tube insertion. He had many health problems and the doctors did not think he would reach eight years old. We were from a small town with an old-fashioned doctor. He instructed us to stop feeding him through the tube and start feeding him by mouth. This is when our journey began with a plant-based diet. They said that he would never walk, he would be in a wheel chair. Praise God, he is not in a wheel chair. He does not talk, but he has his ways of communication. At this time Aaron is twenty-one years old, one hundred forty-five pounds, and six feet two inches tall.

Before there was pain God had a plan. It includes the eight laws of Health.

1. Nutrition - Genesis 1:29 notes how to add vitamins and proteins through vegetables, seeds, nuts, and, Legumes.

2. Exercise - Genesis 2:15 help build blood circulation, weight control and is essential for your heart. A safe way is walking at least 30 minutes a day.

3. Water - Genesis 2:10 The human body is mostly water. An adequate amount of water for proper function is eight to ten glasses a day depending on your activity, size and weight.

4. Sunshine - Genesis 1:3-4 Ten minutes of sunshine each day assists the body to synthesize its own vitamin D.

5. Temperance - 1 Corinthians 9:25 Self-control means not over indulging in anything good or bad for the body. This includes sleeping, eating, exercising, and too much sunlight.

6. Air - Genesis 2:7 Breathe good pure air. Deep breathing clears the mind, helps with depression, improves the digestion system, clears the lungs, and helps with sleeping. Take ten deep breaths at least twice a day.

7. Rest – Exodus 20:8-11 A worn out feeling can be helped greatly simply by resting and proper sleep.

While sleeping the brain cells build up the supply of energy in the body. The body should also have periods of relaxation or a change of activity during the day. Take one day out of the seven days of the week for complete rest and reset. Spiritual fellowship and family togetherness were God's plan from the beginning of creation.

8. Trust in Divine Power - Proverb 3:5, 8 Faith and trusting God's power contributes to remarkable health. God gives the power and self-control needed for a happy life style. Fear and negative emotions slow down and stop the progress of healing. The Lord said that He wishes above all things that man proposer and be in good health 3 John 1:2.

Part One:

What's on the Menu When God Sets the Table?

To answer this question, we must go back. Back to the Garden of Eden when God created us a little over 6,000 years ago. The Bible mentions two very specific interactions between God and humans. Instances when the Creator made decisions based on what He knew to be best instead of compromising in order to accommodate a whining, angry, clueless mob or individual.

This took place soon after Adam and Eve came into existence. God was acting as tour guide to the perfect couple, showing them around their newly created home. The scenery where God planned for Adam and Eve and their descendants to eat, be fruitful, and increase in number. Filling the earth and subduing it. Ruling over the fish of the sea, birds of the air, and all living creatures that move on the ground.

Then the Creator opened the doors of the Eden Garden. "I give you every seed-bearing plant on the face of the whole earth, every tree that has fruit with seeds in it. They will be yours for food." (Genesis 1:29) This may be shocking. God's next statement in Genesis 1 reads like this, "And to all the beasts of the earth and all the birds of the air and all the creatures that move on the ground, everything that has the breath of life in it, I give every green plant for food." (Genesis 1:30) God gave this command because God cared a great deal about what Adam and Eve and their descendants were to eat.

Human bodies are built up from the food taken in. There is a constant breaking down of the tissues of the body. Every movement of every organ of the body requires its share of nutrition. The brain must be supplied with its portion. The bones, muscles, and nerves demand theirs. It is a wonderful process that transforms the food into blood, and this blood builds up the varied parts of the body. This process is going on continually, supplying with life and strength each nerve, muscle, and tissue. *(Ministry of Healing p. 295).*

Those foods should be chosen that best supply the elements needed for building up the body. In order to know what are the best foods one must study God's original plan for man's diet. He who created man and understands his needs appointed Adam's food. *(Counsels on Diet and Foods p. 81).*

Upon leaving Eden to gain his livelihood by tilling the earth under the curse of sin, man received permission to eat also the herbs of the fields. *(Genesis 3:18) (Counsels on Diet and Foods p. 81).*

Foods for Life

Grains, fruits, nuts, and vegetables constitute the diet chose for mankind by the Creator. These foods prepared in as simple and natural a manner as possible are the most healthful and nourishing. They impart strength, power of endurance, vigor of intellect that is not afforded by a more complex and stimulating diet. The diet appointed man in the beginning did not include animals until after the flood when every green thing on the earth had been destroyed, man received permission to eat flesh. *(Counsels on Diet and Foods p. 81).*

In choosing man's food in Eden, the Lord showed what the best diet was. In the choice made for Israel He taught the same lesson. When He brought the Israelites out of Egypt and undertook their training, that they might be a people for His own possession. Through them He desired to bless and teach the world. He provided them with the food best adapted for this purpose, not flesh, but manna, "the bread of heaven." It was because of their murmuring for the fleshpots of Egypt that animal food was granted them, and this only for a short time. This brought disease and death to thousands, because of its use, yet the restriction to a nonflesh diet was never heartily accepted. It continued to cause the discontent and the murmuring, open or secret, and it was not made permanent. *(Counsels on Diet and Foods p. 374).*

In Canaan, the Israelites were permitted to use of animal food but under careful restrictions. No swine's flesh, unclean animal, birds and fish that was pronounced unclean, no fats and blood. All were strictly forbidden. Only animals that as were in good condition, not torn, or died of itself, blood must be carefully drained. *(Counsels on Health and Healing p. 174).*

The knowledge that man is to be a temple for God's habitation for the revealing of His glory, should be the highest incentive to the care and development of our physical powers. *(Ministry of Healing p. 271)*

Part Two:

Has God Changed His Laws?

Some Christians claim God's Law has been changed or done away with. Moses told the Israelites to "Love the Lord, and to keep His charge, His statutes, His judgments, and His commandments always." (Deuteronomy 11:1). Keeping God's Laws would help them to remember who He was and what He had done for them. In this way, they would avoid pain, suffering and sin. What about now? The laws of God are as valid today as in the beginning. It has never changed. There are still ten pillars that embody our relationship with God and the rest of humanity. Nothing has changed except time and culture. The law has not changed nor our need for its guidance.

We cannot keep ourselves from sin for one moment. Every moment we are dependent upon God. For every soul struggling to rise from a life of sin to a life of purity, the great element of power abides in the only name under heaven given among men, whereby we must be saved (Acts 4:12). Christ says, "let him come unto Me and drink."
(John 7:37 last part)

Nothing less than perfect obedience can meet the standard of God's requirement. Christ overcame all the temptations of Satan. By the Word of God, He received power to obey God's commandments, and the tempter could gain no advantage.

Let it be made plain, that the way of God is the way of life. God has established the Laws of Nature, but His laws are not arbitrary exactions. Every "thou shalt not" whether in physical or in moral law, implies a promise. If one will obey it, blessing will attend one's steps. God never forces humanity to do right, but He seeks to save them from the evil and lead them to good. Let attention be called to the laws that were taught to Israel. God gave them definite instruction in regard to their habits of life.

He made known to them the law as relating to both physical and spiritual well-being and on condition of obedience, He assured them. "The Lord will take away from thee all sickness" (Deuteronomy 7:15). "Set your hearts unto all the words which I testify among you this day" (Prov. 4:22), for they are life unto those that find them, and health to all flesh.

Does God Really Care What People Eat?

The desire of God for every human being is expressed in the Words of John "Beloved, I wish above all things that thou mayest prosper and be in health, even as thy soul prospereth," (3 John 2).

"Sickness, suffering, and death are work of an antagonistic power. Satan is the destroyer, God is the restorer. When one recovers from disease, it is God who restores him. All life-giving power is from God. Through the agencies of nature God is working day by day, hour by hour, moment by moment, to keep us alive, to build up and restore. When any part of the body sustains injury, a healing process is at once begun, Nature's agencies are set at work to restore soundness but the power walking through these agencies is the power of God." *(He Cares for Us Every Minute, June 8)*

As stated before it is made plain, that the way of God's commandments is the way of life that God has established in the laws of nature. If people obey its blessing will attend human kind's steps, God never forces them to do right, but He seeks to save them from the evil and lead them to the good.

He calls upon humanity to make choices on the right side, to connect with heavenly agencies to adopt principles of life. It is their work to obtain knowledge of these principles, and by obedience to cooperate with Him in restoring health to the body as well as to the soul. *(Ministry of Healing p. 55)*

Disease never comes without a cause. The way is prepared and disease invited by transgression of sin. The greater number, however; suffer because of their own wrong cause of action. They disregard the principles of health by their habits of eating, drinking, dressing, and working. Their transgressing of nature's laws produces the sure result and when sickness comes upon them, many do not credit their suffering to the true cause, but murmur against God because of their affliction that follows disregard of natural law. Some wish that an exact rule could be prescribed for their diet. They overeat, and then regret it, and so they keep thinking about what they eat and drink. This is not as it should be. One person cannot lay down an exact rule for another. *(Ministry of Healing p. 234)*

Human bodies are Christ's purchased possession and are not at liberty to do with them as they please. (1 Cor. 6:19-20) All who understand the laws of health know they are to be made a matter of personal duty. People must individually answer to God for habits and practices. Therefore, the question with is not, what is the world's practice? But how shall as an individual treat the habitation that God has given? Choose the best food.

Does God really care what humans eat? The diet appointed man in the beginning did not include animal food. It was not until after the flood, when every green thing on the earth had been destroyed, that man received permission to eat flesh.

In choosing man's food in Eden, (Exodus 16:3) the Lord showed what the best diet for man was; in the choice made for Israel, He taught the same lesson. He brought the Israelites out of Egypt and took on their training so that they would be a people for His own possession. Through them, He desired to bless and teach the world. He provided them with the food best adapted for this purpose, not flesh, but manna, the bread of heaven. It was only because of their discontentment and murmuring for the fleshpot of Egypt, that animal food was granted them, and this only for a short time. Its use brought disease and death to thousands. Yet, the restriction to a non-flesh diet was never heartily accepted. It continued to be the cause of discontentment and murmuring, open or secret, and it was not made permanent.

Upon their settlement in Canaan, the Israelites were permitted the use of animal food under careful restrictions, which tended to lessen the evil results. No swine flesh was permitted. Also, along with the other animals, birds, and fish whose flesh was pronounced unclean to eat, there was to be no consumption of blood and the fat of any animal.

By departing from the plan divinely appointed for their diet, Israelites suffered great loss. They desired a flesh diet and they reaped its results. They did not reach God's ideal character or fulfill His purposes. The Lord "gave them their requests, but sent leanness into their soul" (Psalm 106:15). Those who eat flesh are but eating grains and vegetables second handed. The life that was in the grains and vegetables passes to the eater; how much better to get it directly by eating the food that God provided for our use. Flesh was never the best food and those who eat flesh foods little know what they are eating. (*Councils on Diets and Foods/Ministry of Healing p. 313)*

God Has an Original Diet

God's original plan for man's diet was foods that fight diseases: "Grains, fruits, nuts, and vegetables constitute the diet chosen for us by our Creator. These foods, prepared in as simple and natural a manner as possible, are the most healthful and nourishing. *Counsels on Diet and Food, p. 313*

Again and again it has been shown that God is trying to lead humans back, step by step, to His original design, --that man should subsist upon the natural products of the earth. – *[Christian*

Temperance and Bible Hygiene, 119] Counsels on Health, 450, 1890.

Among those who are waiting for the coming of the Lord, meat eating will eventually be done away; flesh will cease to form a part of their diet. People should ever keep this end in view, and endeavor to work steadily toward it. *(Counsels on Diet and Food pp 380,381).*

What is God's diet today? As in the human race disease in animals is increasing, contaminated meat, dairy products, and eggs are common sources of food related illness. "Disease in cattle is making meat eating a dangerous matter. The Lord's curse is upon the earth, upon man, upon beasts, upon the fish in the sea; and as transgression becomes almost universal, the curse will be permitted to become as broad and as deep as the transgression. Disease is contracted by the use of meat." *Counsels on Diet and Food p. 411.* In a short time, it will not be safe to use anything that comes from the animal creation.

The Diet in Eden

After God created the first parents "So God created man in His own image, in the image of God created He him; male and female created He them." Genesis 1:27, He gave them a tour showing them around their newly created home and opened the doors to their Eden Grocery Store. He said to Adam and Eve "Behold, I have given you every herb bearing seed, which is upon the face of all the earth, and every tree, in which is the fruit of a tree yielding seed; to you it shall be for meat." Genesis 1:29. He could have told Adam to pick his own food or asked him what do you want to eat? God knew what was good for man because He had made him. So, He gave him a plant-based diet.

The Diet After the Fall of Man

The fall of man, or man becoming a sinner, happened when man listened to another's voice as it relates to diet. This is recorded in Genesis 3:17-19. It states, "And unto Adam He said, Because thou has hearkened unto the voice of thy wife, and hast eaten of the tree, of which I commanded thee, saying, Thou shalt not eat of it: cursed is the ground for thy sake; in sorrow shalt thou eat of it all the days of thy life; Thorns also and thistles shall it bring forth to thee; and thou shalt eat the herb of the field; In the sweat of thy face shalt you eat bread, till thou return unto the ground; for out of it was thou taken; for dust thou art, and unto dust shalt thou return." So here is shown that God added herbs to the original diet.

The Diet After the Flood

When God had to destroy the earth the first time, he provided for man to eat meat following the flood. He made provision for animal food when God told Noah to take two of every unclean animal, male and female, into the ark but of the clean animals, God told him to take seven, male and female, into the ark. See: "Of every clean beast thou shalt take to thee by sevens, the male and his female: and beasts that are not clean by two, the male and his female. Of fowls also of the air by sevens, the male and the female; to keep seed alive upon the face of all the earth." Genesis 7:2-3. However; in the allowing of flesh food, blood was not included in the diet. Shown in Genesis 9:4 "But the flesh with the life thereof, which is the blood thereof, shall ye not eat." Even the eating of clean bloodless meat had serious consequences. The Bible records a marked decrease in the life span of the post flood patriarchs. "After the flood the people ate largely of animal food. God saw that the ways of man were corrupt, and that he was disposed to exalt himself proudly against his Creator and to follow the inclinations of his own heart. And He permitted that long-lived race to eat animal food to shorten their sinful lives. Soon after the flood the race began to rapidly decrease in size, and in length of years."—*Spiritual Gifts 4a:120-121, 1864.*

The Ideal Diet for Israel

The Israelites were permitted to eat of clean animals [Leviticus 11]. However; they were instructed to eat neither the fat nor the blood. "It shall be a perpetual status for your generations throughout all your dwellings, that ye eat neither fat nor blood," (Leviticus 3:17). In the New Testament, the Gentiles were told to abstain from things strangled and from blood. Acts 15:29. God's ideal diet for Israel is given in Exodus Chapter 16. "Then said the Lord unto Moses, Behold, I will rain bread from heaven for you; and the people shall go out and gather a certain rate every day, that I may prove them, whether they will walk in my law, or not... And the children of Israel did eat manna forty years, until they came to a land inhabited; they did eat manna, until they came unto the borders of the land of Canaan." Exodus 16:4, 35. When God led the children of Israel out of Egypt, it was His purpose to establish them in the land of Canaan a pure, happy, healthy people. He removed flesh food from them in a great measure. "Had they been willing to deny appetite in obedience to His restrictions, feebleness and disease would have been unknown among them.

Their descendants would have possessed physical and mental strength. They would have had clear perceptions of truth and duty, keen discrimination, and sound judgment." *(Counsels on Diet and Food, p. 377-378).*

Daniel's Diet

Daniel and his friends stand out as Biblical examples of the benefits of a temperate healthful flesh-free diet. Daniel requested that they be given pulse (beans) and water for ten days. This simple diet provided not only physical benefits and also mental advantages; "and in all matters of wisdom and understanding, that the king enquired of them, he found them ten times better than all the magicians and astrologers that were in all his realm." Daniel 1:20. Daniel stood out in wisdom, God's wisdom.

Meat Eating Especially Dangerous Now

Flesh was never the best food; but its use is now doubly objectionable, since disease in animals is so rapidly increasing—*The Ministry of Healing, 313, 1905.* Animals are becoming more and more diseased, and it will not be long until animal food will be discarded by many besides Seventh-day Adventist. *Testimonies for the Church Volume 7, p. 124, 1902.*

When will those who know the truth take their stand on the side of right principles for time and for eternity? When will they be true to the principles of health reform? When will they learn that it is dangerous to use flesh meat? If ever meat eating were safe, it is not safe now. *—Manuscript 133, 1902.*

The very animals whose flesh people eat are frequently so diseased that, if let alone, they would die of themselves; but while the breath of life is in them, they are killed and brought to market. People take directly into their system tumors and poison of the worst kind, and yet they realize it not. *Testimonies for the Church Volume 2, pp 404-405.*

Those who use flesh foods little know what they are eating. People are continually eating flesh that is filled with tuberculosis and cancerous germs. *—The Ministry of Healing, 313, 1905.*

A well-balanced diet is most important in maintaining good health. The body can only use the materials we supply from our tables for rebuilding damaged tissues and replacing worn-out parts. If we neglect our diet, we do so at our peril. There is no substitute for a well-balanced system of living. The best vitamins in the world cannot take the place of a sensible diet. It is most important for us to choose our foods wisely and well.

There are other advantages in following a well-planned program of living. Such a diet often costs less than one that leaves a person half-starved of the essential nutrients so needed by the body. In addition, it gives strength and vitality to the whole being, replacing the worn-out cells and restoring the energy that may have been depleted. The most important of all of nature's remedies is a Trust in Divine Power.

As one of the great philosophers said, "I dress his wounds, God healed him". This is just as true today as it was centuries ago. Those who are sick must realize that beyond our best efforts there is always a higher Court of Appeal.

Part Three:

Herbs Created for Man's Use

Genesis 1:29 "Behold I have given you every herb bearing seed, which is upon the face of the earth." The Bible refers to herbs more than three thousand times. Many are mentioned by name and are intended for use. How should herbs be used? The most common herbs are very beneficial when used in combinations.

The Herb Encyclopedia

There is no longer needed extensive research necessary for using nature's medicines.

Alfalfa is a member of the legume family. It is recommended for its bodily influence alternatives. Anodyne, antipyretic, anti-rheumatic, anti-scorbutic, aperitif, depurative, diuretic are all helped by the use of alfalfa. Parts of herb used are the seed and sprout. Good for upset stomachs, the leaves have eight essential amino acids, good for coughs, poultice, earaches, kidney disorders; it is called the "father of all herbs." It has Vitamin C, K, E, and U, which prevents ulcers. It is high in calcium and is the basis for liquid chlorophyll with a balance of chemicals and minerals is used therapeutically for arthritis, a wide range of intestinal and skin disorders, liver problems, breath and body odor, even cancer. Eating any of the green super foods is like giving a transfusion to help treat illnesses, enhance immunity and sustain well-being. Alfalfa contains all the known vitamins and minerals for life. Alfalfa is not a perfect food because it does not contain enough of these nutrients or carbohydrates in high enough amounts to sustain life by just eating Alfalfa.

Alfalfa roots extend deep into the soil where it reaches mineral rich soil, which gives it a high nutrient value. Its roots have been found to come through the tops of the coal miner's tunnels. It is one of the highest chlorophyll bearing plants known to man. Religious groups have used chlorophyll in place of blood transfusions. It is a rich source of B-12, sodium fluoride, a high natural source of Vitamin A. It helps with arthritis, asthma, blood purifier, boils, bursitis, diabetes, flu hemorrhages, gravel, heart disease, tooth decay, and morning sickness.

Others: The high enzymes content of fresh or freeze-dried helps the body to balance its systems, enabling it to ward off infectious disease; even helps to restore the body's immune system. *Herbal Medicine Handbook*

The Lord has given some simple herbs of the field that at times are beneficial and if every family were educated in how to use these herbs in case of sickness, much suffering might be prevented. *EGW, Letter 82 - 1892*

Borage is a body cleanser and blood purifier. It can be used to bathe sore eyes and strengthens the heart. It is also good for coughs by loosening the phlegm.

Chamomile is an excellent general tonic. Chamomile helps to promote appetite and is good for nervous headaches and weak stomachs. It makes a delicious tea mixed with other herbs such as spearmint and clover. It helps regulate monthly periods, helps with colds, kidneys, eye wash and for swelling. It can be made into a poultice.

Catnip can be used as follows: It quiets the nerves, helps infant colic, soothes pain in general, calms stomach acid and bowels. Made into a tea it can be used as an enema for fevers. This process also expels worms. Crush the leaves or juice for skin rashes and skin poisoning.

Coriander is a good stomach tonic. It strengthens the heart and will help to expel gas from the bowels. Coriander also has a good flavor and helps when used with unpleasant tasting herbs.

Corn silk increases the flow of urine. It relieves pain and inflammation in the kidney, bladder and prostate gland. It is excellent for prevention of bed wetting. It is used by making a strong tea from it.

Charcoal has many benefits. Use olive oil and stir in a little charcoal and take for indigestion. It can also be mixed with soybean milk and taken for indigestion. It is good for cleansing and healing. The best charcoal is from shells of coconut, willow, soft pine wood, and eucalyptus trees. Charcoal is good for fomentation, heartburn, gas, cleaning teeth, snake bites, insect bites, sores and bruises, inflamed eyes, when used as a poultice. It is very beneficial when taken after a meal. Use 1 teaspoon mixed with water and drink.

For catarrh, coughs and asthma use comfrey. Taken as a tea, comfrey is helpful to relieve diarrhea, anemia, and female debility. It can also be used as a poultice and applied to sore breasts, wounds, burns, and sores.

Fennel is a wonderful herb for flavoring foods. It can be used as medicine too. Fennel is a good remedy for indigestion, gas, acid stomach, cramps and colic. Sprinkle fennel on food and soups. It can be used in beans to prevent gas. Steeped in boiling water fennel makes a wonderful tea using fresh leaves or seeds. Fennel has a refreshing taste and will make the breath sweeter. Fennel is an old household remedy found in almost every Italian garden

Flaxseed is a common seed and is used on cereal. It is usually ground and can be in water and jellied, whipped stiff like egg whites. It is used in the place of egg for those who prefer plant foods only. Flaxseeds can be made into a thick mush by mixing with hot water. This forms a poultice and mixed with other herbs it can be used for boils, sores, tumors and carbuncles. Flaxseed is a wonderful food for the hair. It is high in unsaturated fats.

Golden Seal is an extremely bitter but the most wonderful herb remedy in the herb kingdom. It is a body cleanser, tonic, laxative, can be used for cleansing wounds, helps with ulcers, bathing the eyes, used as an antiseptic, colds, stomach and liver troubles. Golden seal is most helpful for mucous membranes, skin diseases and can be used internally and externally. It is good for chronic catarrhal conditions. Golden Seal will improve the appetite and aid indigestion. Mixed with myrrh and other herbs it is excellent in many ways. Some have called it a "cure all."

Hops induces sleep. It is a sedative. It has an efficient quieting effect. It helps in delirium tremors, toothaches, boils, tumors, and excessive sexual desires. It can be made into a poultice and placed over the stomach to relieve pain. For sleep, drink two cups of hot tea.

Hyssop is an old Biblical remedy. Hyssop, in connection with the proper use of water and deep breathing, is a wonderful body cleanser for children's diseases, sore throat and phlegm in the lungs and throat. It is good for circulation. It is a fine tonic for weakened conditions and for fevers. For best results steep one teaspoon of hyssop in one cup of boiling water for twenty minutes.

Lavender is a flower that is used in making perfumes and is often dried and put in drawers and linen closets to make them smell good; however, it also has an excellent culinary use. When used as a tea, lavender is a good tonic and prevents faintness and stops nausea. When combined with other herbs it can overpower bad taste of the other herbs and is a great seasoning.

Marjoram is very effective in combination with chamomile to assist with sour stomach issues. It can also be used to aid with the loss of appetite. Another wonderful use of marjoram is to suppress problems in menstruations as well as assist with headache and indigestion. Taken hot will produce perspiration.

Mustard powder is excellent to put in hot foot bath for congestion and colds. It draws blood to the lower part of the body. Use one part mustard and two parts whole wheat flour mixed to make an excellent plaster. When mixed with egg whites, it can be used to prevent blistering.

Peppermint and **Spearmint** should be in every garden. They are an excellent remedy for colds, chills, colic, dizziness, fevers, gas in the stomach, nausea, vomiting, headache, diarrhea and flu. Peppermint or spearmint can be used externally and applied for relief in rheumatism. Peppermint is a wonderful natural stimulant. When combined with other herbs. Peppermint and spearmint make a refreshing drink. The differences in the appearance of the two herbs: the leaves of the peppermint are broader, shorter, and darker shade of green than that of the spearmint.

Plantain is a small wild plant with leaves that grow mainly from the plant's base. The flowers are tiny, greenish, and in spikes. It's native to northern temperate regions and belongs to the family of Plantaginaceae. There are two kinds of plantains, narrow and wide leaf. Both are good. The whole plant should be used. Fresh crushed leaves give quick relief when rubbed on poison ivy and insect bites. Rub whole leaves on piles or hemorrhoids and rectal itching. This will give quick relief. The fresh leaves pounded into a paste are good applied to sores and ulcers. It can also be applied to wounds and will check bleeding when used for piles and hemorrhoids. Plantain can be made into a tea. Make into a strong tea and place in syringe and apply to piles and hemorrhoids. The plant can also be boiled in olive oil for about an hour, strained and use for skin rash and healing of other sores.

Raspberry is helpful during pregnancy. It makes childbirth wonderfully easy. It is an old Indian remedy. Raspberry is a good remedy for painful menstruation. The herb Spikenard can also be used in such cases. It is a wonderful blood purifier.

Red Clover is a wonderful blood purifier. It may be taken as freely as water and is very soothing to the nerves. This herb is effective in whooping cough. Drink freely on empty stomach or bathe sores with tea. The blossoms can be gathered in the summer. Dry them and store in clean quart jars.

Rosemary is an old fashion remedy for colds and nervous conditions. Make a tea of the herb and drink warm. It is a good mouth wash for gums and aids in bad breath and sore throat. It is a good stomach remedy and aids in digestion.

Sage is wonderful for coughs, colds, mucous, asthma, fevers, and tonsillitis. Gargle with a strong tea and swallow some. It is good for nervous headaches and will dry up milk when nursing.

Sassafras is a good spring cleaner to purify the blood and cleanse the entire system. It is a good remedy for spasms and will relieve gas. Sassafras is a good skin remedy and is good for toothache. Using sassafras helps to give other disagreeable herbs a better taste. It can be used as a substitute for cinnamon. Combine it with Anise and Coriander.

Sorrel used as a green is very high in nutritive properties. When it is ground fine, it makes a wonderful addition to soybean curd mixed with a little mayonnaise. Sorrel is good to expel worms and is warming to the heart. When sorrel is made into a poultice it aids with boils and tumors. The leaves eaten in a salad are an excellent preventive for scurvy.

Thyme is good for fevers (Ma Tea) and will produce perspiration. It is good for nerves when taken hot. Thyme is good to reduce nightmares, whooping cough, and asthma and lung troubles. It relieves headaches in children.

Watermelon Seeds are beneficial in bladder troubles. Make a strong tea by steeping seeds in boiling water.

Wintergreen assists in stomach problems, heart, respiration, colic and gas in bowels. The oil of wintergreen is useful in liniments. The flavor of wintergreen is pleasant especially when honey is added.

Wormwood is used to expel worms, aids with swelling, rheumatism, sprains, and poor digestion.

Part Four:

Super Foods

Aca is a little purple berry. It is loaded with antioxidants that protect from a variety of conditions. It is also known as the Amazonian palm berry. It grows on large palm trees, the same trees that produce Hearts of Palm. It tastes like a mix of chocolate and berry. This antioxidant fight against heart disease.

Green and blue-green algae are phytoplanktons. They have been called perfect super foods. They have abundant high-quality digestible protein, fiber, chlorophyll, vitamins, minerals and enzymes. They are the most potent source of beta carotene available in the world today; they are the richest food source of vitamin B-12.

Chlorella contains a higher concentration of chlorophyll than any other known plant. It is a complete protein food with all the B vitamins, C and E. It has many minerals and is a high enough source of these vitamins to be considered a supplement.

Spirulina is the original green super food. It is an easily produced algae with the ability to grow in both ocean and alkaline water. Acre for acre, spirulina yield twenty times more protein than soybeans, forty times more protein than corn, and vitamins including B-12. It is rich in beta carotene, minerals, and essential fatty acids.

Barley, Wheatgrass, and Alfalfa are helpful for high blood pressure problems, fatigue, obesity, diabetes, gastritis ulcers, pancreas, and liver problems, asthma, eczema, hemorrhoids, skin problems, anemia, constipation, breath and body odor. They are especially effective for oral inflammations, bleeding gums, osteomyelitis (chronic bone marrow inflammation) burns, athlete's foot, and cancer. Also good for bones, they are rich sources of vitamin K. They help maintain normal bone metabolism and improve energy.

Barley grass has a wide range of concentrated vitamins, minerals, enzymes, proteins, and chlorophyll. It has eleven times the calcium of cow's milk, five times the iron of spinach, and seven times the amount of vitamin C and bioflavonoid as in orange juice. One of its most important contributions to a vegetarian diet is 80 mg of vitamin B-12 in 100 grams of powdered juice, encouraging results for DNA damage repair and delaying aging. Contains anti-viral properties and neutralizes heavy metals like mercury. It is an ideal food source anti-inflammatory for healing gastro-intestinal ulcers, hemorrhoids, and pancreas infections. Barley grass is an ideal anti-inflammatory medication, stronger than steroids and non-steroid drugs. It has no side effects.

Alfalfa is one of the world's richest mineral sourced foods pulling up earth minerals from the roots depths as great as 130 feet. It is an excellent source for liquid chlorophyll with a balance of organic chemical and mineral consistent almost identical to human hemoglobin. It is a body cleanser, infection fighter, a natural deodorizer, it has a rich source of fiber and good spring tonic, eliminates retained water, relieves urinary and bowel problems, helping to treat cases of narcotic and alcohol addiction. It is used therapeutically for arthritis, intestinal and skin disorders for blood clotting, because of its high content of Vitamin K. it is also used to treat bladder infection, anemia, hemorrhaging, diabetes, and aids in normalizing estrogen production.

Wheatgrass has curative powers for treating cancerous growths and other degenerative diseases. Fifteen pounds of fresh liquid has the nutritional value of three hundred fifty pounds of vegetables. There has been particular success with wheatgrass rectal implants in colon cancer cases. Wheatgrass helps cleanse the blood, organs, and gastrointestinal tract, and is recommended as a way to stimulate metabolism and enzyme activity. It also normalizes the thyroid gland, strengthen cells, detoxifies the liver and blood and chemically neutralize pollutant. It also helps to resist harm from the destructive effects of air pollution, ex-rays, radiation and especially carbon monoxide.

Aloe Vera is known as an effective skin moisturizer and healer for cuts, sunburns, bruises, insect bites, skin sores, acne, eczema, and burns in gel form. Aloe juice is now becoming widely known for its digestive, soothing laxative properties, specific for colon problems and liver diseases. Aloe has excellent trans-dermal properties, allowing it to penetrate deep skin levels, pre-op and post-op, it is a natural antiseptic, astringent for infection, both internal and external it is a natural oxygenator, increasing the body intake of oxygen, for arthritis, skin cancer, hemorrhoids, and varicose veins. Aged Aloe Vera juice is even being widely used in Aids Treatment to block the HIV virus movement from cell to cell. One of the best colon cleansers. Its common names are Bomba Aloe, Turkey Aloe, and Mocha Aloe. *(Back to Eden. Pg. 197-198).*

Iodine and Healing

Iodine is essential to life since the thyroid gland cannot regulate metabolism without it. It is an important element of alertness and rapid brain activity. In this era of processed foods and iodine poor soils, sea vegetables and sea foods stand almost alone as potent sources of natural balanced iodine.

Iodine is also a key factor in the control and prevention of many endocrine deficiency conditions prevalent today; such as breast and uterine fibroid tumors, prostate inflammation, toxic liver and kidney problems. Thyroid hormones are made from iodine and the amino acid tyrosine. Iodine deficiency results in the development of goiter and enlarged thyroid gland. When the level of the iodine is low in the diet and blood, it causes the thyroid gland to become quite large due to pituitary stimulation. Sea vegetables have the ability to reduce tumors, to lower serum cholesterol, and to aid metabolism and digestion.

Foods that are high in iodine include "Seaweed, which is a good source of antioxidants, vitamins and minerals. It is one of the best natural sources of iodine. Three popular seaweed varieties include kombu kelp, wakame and nori. Kombu Kelp is a brown seaweed sold dried or as a fine powder. It can contain up to 2,984 mcg of iodine per seaweed sheet (1 gram). This provides almost 2,000% of the recommended daily intake. Wakame is another type of brown seaweed that is slightly sweet in flavor. It is commonly used to make miso soup. Nori is a type of red seaweed. Unlike brown seaweeds, it has a much lower content of iodine. Nori is the type of seaweed that is commonly used in sushi rolls." *Kaitlyn Berkheiser, Healthline, February 2, 2018.*

Prunes are plums that have been dried. Prunes are a good source of iodine. "Prunes are packed with vitamins and nutrients. Five dried prunes provide a good vegetarian source of iodine by meeting 9% of the daily value." *Ibid February 2, 2018.*

Other fruits and vegetables that contain iodine; however, the concentration of iodine will vary are: lima beans, carrots, bananas, cucumber, sweet pepper, round tomato, cherry tomato, baked potato with peel, and navy beans.

Some vegetables such as broccoli and cabbage are full of fiber and other nutrients but they may interfere with the production of thyroid hormone if you have an iodine deficiency. *Healthline January 30, 2020*

Part Five:

Nature's Own Remedies

In addition to all the wonderful new medicines now available, there are certain natural remedies that everyone can and should use. These are Sunlight, fresh Air, pure Water, Rest, Exercise, a well-balanced diet, and Trust in Divine Power. They are all available at almost no cost.

Sunlight is for toning up the skin and keeping germs under control, when combined with fresh pure air. Pure water is needed to keep the body machinery operating smoothly and efficient at all times. Rest and exercise are equally important in our modern age. The person who is wise will take sufficient exercise at all times so that both mind and body are kept in the best of conditions. Years ago, there was much virtue in people having to work with their hands, spinning and weaving, planting and building, harvesting and drawing water by hand. Today, when so much is provided without effort, one can become weakened through not using the muscles of the body. At the same time, the mind may be over stimulated by emotion packed programs so that adequate rest at night is well-nigh impossible. Be sure to get adequate rest each day so that both mind and body are kept in the best condition at all times.

Arthritis

Arthritis is a catchall term that includes rheumatism (inflammation or pain in muscles, joints, or fibrous tissue) bursitis (inflammation of shoulder, elbow, or knee joint) and gout (joint inflammation caused by an excess of uric acid in the blood). Some Specialists believe that arthritis is a form of rheumatism. Still others claim there is no ailment as rheumatism. That it is a term for several diseases, including arthritis. No matter what it's called, everyone agrees on two things - the pain and that all these conditions involve inflammation of connective tissue of one or more joints, according to the U.S. Centers for Disease Control and Prevention in Atlanta (Health Resource on page 309) for more information. Learn about nonchemical and low-acid diets. There are foods that have been classified as nightshade foods; white potatoes, eggplants, green peppers, and tomatoes are the most common ones that may contribute to the pain of some arthritis sufferers.

Remedies

Cherries help prevent crystallization of uric acid, and reduce the levels of uric acid in the blood. Fresh string beans every day or juice; drink a glass of juice daily. They contain vitamins A, B-12, B-2, and C, which help to relieve the excess acid; one half cup of parsley before breakfast, dinner, and one-half cup anytime pain is particularly severe. Celery contains much organic sulfur. Celery has the power to help neutralize uric acid and other excess acids in the body. The leaves of the celery are also good to eat.

Atherosclerosis

Atherosclerosis is clogging of the arteries that caused by deposits of fatty substances, cholesterol, calcium, and other matter. This build up is called plaque, and it develops over many years from poor diet, a sedentary lifestyle and smoking. It's important that you work with your doctor. Be sure to consult him/her before trying any natural remedies.

Remedies

Eating a few cloves of garlic each day has been known to help clear arteries. It seems to cleanse the system and collect and cast out toxic waste. Mince two cloves and put them in a half glass of orange juice or water and drink it down. No need to chew the piece of garlic.

Back Pain

Lumbago/Herniated Disc/Scoliosis

Common symptoms include spinal stress and pain, the inability to do even small bending or pushing actions and sometimes inability to move at all.

Common causes: Poor posture, improper lifting, or standing, arthritis, deep-seated-emotional stress, kidney malfunction, usually from dehydration, wearing high heels, being overweight, too much protein and calcium.

Diet

The diet should be high in minerals and vegetable proteins. Vegetarians are able to fight plaque because of the phytochemicals in their diet. Reduce the fat in your diet; the greater the deposits of fatty plaque, the greater the degeneration of spinal discs. Green drink is for absorbable minerals and chlorophyll strength. A protein drink like green smoothie is the perfect meal. Hops or Comfrey tea, castor oil pack, cayenne, ginger heat packs, aloe gel, ginger gel, and chamomile oil.

Bone Health

Healing bone breaks, preventing brittle bones, and cartilage re-growth is possible. Continuing research is showing that several common medications put bone health at risk.

Common symptoms: Brittle bones with easy bone breakage, poor bone healing, prematurely gray hair (before 40) is sometimes a sign of decreased bone, mineral mass.

Common causes: Mineral deficiency or poor bone assimilation, poor diet with too many refined foods and too much protein, causing phosphorus imbalance: enzyme deficiency; heavy metal or drug toxicity steroids.

Diet

Maintain a mineral-rich vegetable protein diet helps ratify the condition. Love your liver, keep it healthy. Avoid all refined foods. Acid forming foods like fried and fast foods and cola drinks and sugar inhibits calcium absorption; caffeine causes a loss of calcium. Salt decreases bone density. You may have prematurely gray hair so you may have decreased mineral bone mass for calcium and silicon. The use of sea vegetables, whole grain, tofu, yogurt, for bone; dried fruits, nuts and seeds, honey is helpful for overall health. For Vitamin C, papayas, kiwi, strawberry, bell peppers, broccoli, and cantaloupe. Also, nutritional yeast, miso, beta carotene, Vitamin K, aloe live, aloe gold, Bilberry, nettles, and ginseng.

Asthma

A breathing disorder that is on a 50% rise from 1985 to 1995. Common symptoms: difficult breathing, choking, wheezing, coughing, difficulty in exhaling, often with heart palpitations. Colds are often accompanied by ear infections, a croupy cough accompanying hyperactivity in kids, high blood pressure in adults.

Common causes: Food allergies, particularly to additives or preservatives, excess sugar, pasteurized dairy products, meats, wheat. Adrenal exhaustion and imbalance, hypoglycemia, poor circulation and constipations, an increased toxic food from chemical environmental pollutants, sprayed produce, emotional stress, or excessively cold air, low thyroid and adrenal exhaustion. Diet improvement is the key factor for maintaining control of asthma.

Diet

Green leafy veggies provide needed magnesium. Garlic juice, cayenne, olive oil and honey, mix then take one teaspoon daily as a liver cleansing bile stimulant for fatty acid metabolism. Aloe, green supreme, Ginkgo Biloba, Reish, Lobelia, as a chest muscle relaxant, and mushroom capsules are also good to aid in control of the condition. Apply an onion poultice or hot ginger compress to the chest. Use Vitamin E 400 IU.

Cataracts

Macular Degeneration Lens Opacity: Cataracts are the leading cause of impaired vision in America, affecting over a four million people.

Cataract surgery is the most common operation for people over 65 performed over million times a year.

Common symptoms: Cataracts appear as cloudy or opaque areas on the crystalline lens of the eye which focuses light they block light entering the eyes. Macular degeneration: blurry, distorted vision, decreased reading ability, even with large type, faded colors glasses do not help. Driving is very difficult because of blind spots.

Common causes of cataracts: Free radical damage, from heavy metal/environmental pollutants or UV rays. Too much dietary fats, sugar, salt, and cholesterol; linked to diabetes, poor circulation and constipation, liver malfunction, protein deficiency with poor enzyme activity. Macular degeneration, poor digestion, linked to UV sunlight. People with light colored eyes are more at risk.

Diet

Reduce intake of fats, cholesterol foods, blood sugar stability is a key factor. Include green leafy veggies, celery, citrus fruits, brewer's yeast, sprouts, apples and apple juice; add legumes for sulfur, containing amino acids, and carrots juice, daily for three months. Eat lutein rich foods especially kale, collard greens, and spinach, whole grains, beans, and pumpkin seeds, aloe vera juice. Use as eye drops two times daily, without ascorbic acid, eyebright eyewash, rosehips eyewash, Ginkgo Biloba extra caps four times daily, Bilberry tea Ginkgo Biloba extract, Chamomile, wear amber or blue blocking sunglasses, especially when driving.

Carpal Tunnel Syndrome

Repetitive Strain Injury

While Carpal Tunnel Syndrome has long been a problem for knitters and needle workers, and those doing repetitive task jobs, such as carpenters, musicians and assembly-line workers, it is a common ailment of the computer age affecting more than one out of ten Americans who work on computers. Standard medical treatment is usually cortisone shots to control swelling. In severe cases, surgery to enlarge the carpal tunnel opening is used more and more. Natural therapies can both relieve pain and act as a preventative to the development of C.T.S.

Diet

Eat plenty of fresh foods with at least one green salad every day. Add celery for good cell activity and sea vegetables or miso soup to alkalize the blood. Take a glass of lemon juice and water each morning. Make a mix with two teaspoons each of lecithin granules, brewer's yeast, molasses and toasted wheat germ. Add one tablespoon to the daily diet. Enjoy green drinks, fresh carrot drink, beta carotene drink, fiber and C support drink. Some teas good for the nerve are Skullcap, and Lobelia Ginkgo Biloba. Drink two to three times a day.

Cellulite

Fatty Deposits in the Skin

Cellulite is actually a combination of fat and water and trapped waste beneath the skin. Usually on otherwise thin women. When the body's circulation and elimination process become impaired, tissue loses its strength. Un-metabolized fats and wastes become trapped in the vulnerable cells just beneath the skin instead of being expelled through normal means. Over a period of time, these waste materials harden and form the puckering skin effect we know as cellulite.

Diet

Have a fresh salad every day. Have one or two fresh or steamed vegetables at every meal. Have brown rice once a day. Eat fruits and juices in the morning. Use small amounts of unsaturated oils. Have omega rich sea food twice a week. Have two tablespoons of sea vegetables three or four times a week in a soup or salad. Eat small meals instead of two or three large ones. Drink six to eight glasses of water. Drink Hawthorn extract to reduce blood fat levels and stabilize heart rate. Rub on Rosemary,

Thyme, and Peppermint oil to increase metabolism and to stimulate circulation.

Weight Loss

Excess Fat Retention

Weight loss is a nutritional obsession in America yet 34 million American adults are obese. Another 45 million are overweight (this doesn't count children who are rapidly becoming an overweight generation); 25 million Americans are seriously dieting. As fried foods have increased in our diets and physical labor has decreased, there has been 500-800% increase in obesity in the 20th Century. The answers to weight control aren't simple. The most serious dieters are able to lose about 10% of their body weight on a strict diet, yet two thirds of that weight is gained back within five years. Crash diets, especially those that are almost totally fat-free, are impossible to stick with. It is intolerable for a normal lifestyle and even dangerous to health because they are so imbalanced.

Diet

The four keys to an effective weight control diet are low fat, high fiber, regular exercise, and lots of water. The importance of cutting back on fat cannot be over-stated. Changing diet composition is the passport to weight control. Some helpful herbs are Citrimax with Kelp and Ginseng, Bee Pollen, and for high protein energy, Omega-3 Flax Oil. Wild yam caps for highest natural DHEA, an appetite suppressor.

Taste and Smell Loss

Deviated Septum

There is a broad variety of reasons for this dysfunction, which includes a deviated septum. It does respond to several common drugs people take today for colds and flu. In addition, nerve endings maybe damaged from arthritis or osteoporosis. This is one of the reasons the problem affects older people more than younger. The natural healing emphasis on overcoming nutritional deficiencies is often able to successfully address many of the root causes. If total atrophy has not developed, at least partial taste and smell can be restored.

Common symptoms are the inability or only partial ability to smell odors or taste foods.

Common causes include zinc and other mineral deficiencies, zinc excretion and too many antibiotics. It is a side effect of chemotherapy. Deviated septum, chronic low-grade throat and sinus infection, poor circulation and a mucous clogged system. High blood pressure medicine, cold medicine, and poor hormone secretion all contribute to loss of taste and smell.

Diet

A mineral rich, low fat, low salt, diet is a key factor to help restore normal function of the sense of smell and taste. Keep the diet free of mucous-clogging foods. Add of plenty fresh, crunchy, high texture foods like: celery, apples, and green salads. Everyday include grains, green leafy vegetables, brown rice, miso soup, and sea vegetables. Everyday include Orange Peel Tea, Ginseng drink, Kelp tablets, (six daily), Vitamin B, Alfa juice/caps, chlorophyll, (one teaspoon before meals), this will help restore function as well.

Moles/Warts

Moles are congenital, discolored growths elevated above the skin and may be evidence of a liver or lung condition. They are harmless unless continually irritated.

Warts are single or clustered soft irregular skin growths found on the hands, feet, arms, and face. They range in size from a pinhead to a small bean. They can also occur on the throat or voice box and affect the speaking voice tone. Usually caused by a virus, they are contagious and will spread if picked, bitten, or nicked through shaving.

Common symptoms and appearance of warts and flat or raised modules on the skin surface are a rough pitted discolored surface that sometimes causes pain.

Common Causes are Vitamin A and mineral deficiencies, viral infection, use of antibiotics and vaccinations that depress normal immunity.

Diet

Add Vitamin A rich foods to the diet, such as asparagus, green fruits, garlic, onions, fresh figs, and citrus fruits. Also using Vitamin C foods with bioflavonoid are most potent. Yogurt is also a good source.

Application: Jojoba oil, cinnamon oil, grapefruit seed extract, nettle extract, and garlic oil.

Vertigo

Dizziness/Inner Ear Malfunction/Meniere's Syndrome

Vertigo is a result of equilibrium (inner ear) disturbance with the sensation of moving around in space, or of having objects move around you. It occurs when the brain and central nervous system get conflicting messages from the body sensors that effect and maintain balance, the ear, eyes, and skin pressure receptions.

Common symptoms start with ear pain, ringing and pressure. A feeling of faintness, lightheadedness, and falling or lack of steadiness upon standing up quickly and feeling off balance. Vertigo victims also have frequent hearing loss and nausea.

Common causes: poor circulation and blood pressure imbalance (which shows up if you stand or move to quickly) lack of brain oxygen, or brain tumors, food and chemical allergies, neurological disease, chronic stress, and anxiety hypoglycemia excess ear wax, Vitamin B deficiency.

Diet

The diet should be low in saturated fats and cholesterol, high in vegetable proteins, Vitamin B foods, such as brown rice, broccoli, tofu, seafood, and sprouts, and a green drink daily. Eliminate common allergy foods, wheat, corn, dairy products, sprayed foods like oranges and lettuce, and fried foods.

Mix brewer's yeast and wheat germ (or two teaspoons of wheat germ oil) two tablespoons and use on a fresh salad daily. Drink Butchers Broom Tea, Catnip, St John's Wart, Cayenne, Ginger capsules, Peppermint, if it is nausea. Take Ginseng with honey in water as a daily drink.

Water Retention

Bloating Edema

Water retention, the excessive accumulation of fluid in body tissues and cavities, is often a problem of not enough water; a condition of body imbalance. If we don't get sufficient water, fluid levels go out of balance and the body begins to retain more water in an effort to compensate. Kidney, liver, blood pressure, circulation, pre-menstrual and pregnancy problems, are all associated with water retention. Dieting can take away foods that previously provide water. Medical diuretics, alcoholic drinks, and drugs can dehydrate. A natural healing program should concentrate on balancing body chemistry rather than simply releasing water.

Diet

Reduce salt and salty foods in-take. Eat largely fresh foods for three to five days to increase the body's food water content without density. Have a leafy green salad every day to increase the body's food water. Have plenty cucumbers, parsley, alfalfa sprouts, and celery. Avoid starchy and sugary foods. Reduce dried and dairy foods that demand more water to dissolve. Drink at least six to eight bottles of water daily for free-flowing functions of waste removal and appetite, suppression. Drink diuretic herbal teas, Corn Silk, Dandelion, Juniper, and Parsley.

Varicose Veins

Spider Veins/Peripheral Problem

Peripheral vascular problems like varicose veins are more than a cosmetic nuisance. They can be painful, cause unusual fatigue and heaviness, and leg and ankle swelling, and cramping. Varicose veins develop when a defect in the vein wall causes dilation in the vein and damage to the valves; when the valves are not functioning well, the increased pressure results in bulging. Spider veins are thin, red, unsightly lines on the face, upper arms, and thighs. Women are affected four times as frequently as men. Vein fragility increases with age due to the loss of tissue, tone, muscles mass, and weakening of vein walls.

Common symptoms: Distended swollen, painful, bulging leg veins; the leg will feel heavy, tight, sometimes with numbness and tingling; thin red spider veins, and muscle cramps.

Common causes: Low-fiber diet, dairy based diet, too many refined foods, poor posture and circulation, liver malfunction, long periods of standing, damage to veins from inflammation and blood clots in the vein.

Diet

A high unrefined fiber diet is most beneficial. Go on a 24-hour liquid diet to clear circulation, and then eat only fresh foods for the rest of the week. Follow high fiber vegetarian diet for the rest of the month. Then beans, whole grains cereals, Vitamin C juice daily, pineapple, carrots, cherries, berries, brown rice, grapes, Ginkgo Biloba, Hawthorn extract, Kotu-Kola, Ginger Root, garlic, and onions capsules. All these items will help reverse symptoms and appearance of varicose veins, spider veins, and peripheral problems.

Cholesterol

Hyperlipidemia/High Serum LDL or VLDL/High Triglyceride

Cholesterol is a fat related substance in the body that is needed for many processes related to nerve and hormone functions. Poor metabolism and over-indulgence in high cholesterol foods lead to serious deposits in arterial and linings and to gallstones. There are two kinds of cholesterol [HDL] and [VLDL]. HDL is low density and very low density, lipo-protein or bad cholesterol. Triglycerides are a sugar related blood fat that travels with cholesterol, as lipo-protein. High triglycerides can cause blood cells to stick together impairing circulation leading to heart attack.

Common symptoms: Plaque formation on the arterial walls, poor circulation, legs cramps and pain, high blood pressure, cold hands and feet, dry skin and dizziness, allergies, and kidney trouble.

Common causes: Stress, diet, sugar, saturated fats, and low fiber in the diet.

Diet

A low-fat high fiber diet is the key to reducing cholesterol reducing sugar is the key. Soy foods, olive oil, whole grains, like oats, fruits, and vegetables, yogurt, cultured foods and yams, cayenne/ginger capsules two times a day, garlic tablets six tablets a day, turmeric, and golden seal, and myrrh extract.

Circulation Problems

Sluggish Blood Flow/Claudication/Raynaud's Disease

Sluggish circulation can stem from many body conditions. It transports heat from the inner body to the skin. It carries antibodies to areas of infection. It helps move waste products to channels of elimination. Sluggish circulation is one of the signs of serious disorder. High blood pressure, arteriosclerosis, varicose veins, phlebitis, and heart disease are all connected with circulation system health. Investigate further if your condition does not improve.

Common symptoms: Cold hands and feet, poor memory, migraine headaches, numbness, ringing in the ears and hearing loss, dizziness, shortness of breath, high triglyceride and cholesterol levels.

Common causes: Cholesterol plaque on artery walls, low fiber in diet, constipation, and lack of exercise.

Diet

Eat citrus fruits, juices and dried fruits. Drink plenty of healthy fluids. Eat smaller meals. Mix one half cup tomato juice, one half cup lemon juice, six teaspoons' wheat germ oil, one teaspoon brewer's yeast. Rosemary, Butcher's Broom, Ginseng, Ginkgo Biloba extracts are also helpful.

Colds

Upper Respiratory Infections

The common cold is quite normal during high risk seasons. About a third of America suffers from colds. A cold is usually an attempt by the body to cleanse itself of wastes, toxins, and bacteria, overgrowths that have built up to the point where natural immunity cannot handle or overcome them. The glands are always affected and as the endocrine system is on a six-day cycle, a normal cold usually runs for about a week.

Diet

Go on a liquid diet during acute stage with green or potassium, drink to clean out infection and mucous, eat fresh and steamed vegetables. Fresh fruits and juices teas Echinacea, golden seal capsules, cayenne, and garlic capsules.

Tumors - Malignant

Malignant tumors should be addressed as soon as possible to control spreading to other tissues. Tumors may be internal as brain gland or external organ tumors. Brain tumors especially should be acted upon immediately because both malignant and benign tumors can cause irreversible neurological damage. Brain tumors are likely to return if not completely excised. Immune enhancement is the key in natural treatment. A whole plant food diet is best.

Common symptoms: Growing and mutating lumps and nodules often inflamed, weeping and painful, many times with adhesions to other tissue. Brain tumors include chronic headaches, unexplained vomiting, weakness, and lethargy.

Changes in vision sometimes are accompanied by seizures and stupors.

Common causes: Poor diet, years of excess acid and mucous forming foods, heavy metal or radiation poisoning, x-rays, iodine deficiency.

Diet

Begin with a short liquid cleansing diet; for one month – have one each day: potassium broth, a veggie drink, cranberry, pineapple juice. Then add whole grain, high fiber foods, and steamed vegetables. Keep the system by clean by cleaning the liver. Drink only distilled bottle water about six to eight bottles daily. Add high sulfur foods. Aloe life, aloe Vera juice, garlic/onion capsules, green foods, aloe cold drink, Pau d'Arco, Echinacea, extract of ginseng, six super caps or tea.

Ulcers

Stomach Peptic Duodenal

Approximately 14 million Americans now have or recently had an ulcer. Ten thousand people die of peptic ulcer every year. A peptic ulcer is an open sore, an erosion of the lining either in the stomach (a gastric ulcer) or the duodenum (the first part of the small intestine). Most ulcers are caused by H-pylori, a common stomach bacteria which liberate copious amounts of damaging ammonia and carbon dioxide when the body's intestinal protective devices fail. The use of natural therapy focuses on gastric mucosal support and re-establishing intestinal balance.

Common Causes include mental and emotional stress which creates an acid system. Gastro intestinal irritants like smoking, aspirin, NSAID drugs, coffee, and alcohol, poor food combining and eating too fast, food allergies, too much sugary foods, anemia hypoglycemia contributes as well to ulcers.

Diet

Go on a three-day liquid diet to cleanse and alkalize the GI tract. Take three glasses of your choice juice daily, potassium broth, veggie drink, cabbage, celery, parsley juice, apple, alfalfa sprouts, and raw cabbage salad daily during healing.

Avoid sugars, fatty foods, spice refined foods. Drink teas such as slippery elm, marshmallow root, golden seal, turmeric, chamomile, comfrey, and take cayenne capsules.

Cerebral Palsy

Muscle/Nerve Dysfunction

Cerebral Palsy is the most common crippling childhood disorder. Cerebral is a broad term for brain-centered motor disorders, which usually occur before or during birth. Damage to the cerebrum causes a paralysis (palsy) in one or more parts of the body. The damage is sustained throughout adulthood. Premature infants with low birth weight (less than 3 ½ pounds) are at high risk for developing cerebral palsy, especially if the mother has been addicted to drugs.

Common symptoms of Cerebral Palsy are characterized by a loss of control over voluntary muscles and abrupt jerking muscle contraction. It also involves spastic convulsive seizures and often atrophy of the muscle.

Commonly caused by being passed on hereditary through drug abuse or over-use in the mother, especially when it causes inadequate oxygen supply to the brain. It also causes clogged motor control centers in different locations in the brain due to malnutrition as an infant. It can be caused by infant diseases such as encephalitis meningitis or herpes simplex, heavy meal poisoning, and nerve malfunction through deficient prostaglandin formation.

Diet

A modified macrobiotic diet is effective. Eat organically grown foods as much as possible. Include plenty of leafy greens in the diet with a fresh salad every day.

Go on a cleansing juice fast one day a week until symptoms improve (usually 3-4 months). Take a potassium broth every other day during the cleanse. Avoid refined foods, saturated fats, fried foods, and caffeine.

Make a mix with 2 tablespoons each of brewer's yeast, lecithin, and toasted wheat germ. Take some daily over cereal or in juice. Take Nutritional yeast or miso in water before bed. The teas to use are Gotu Kola, bilberry, ginger, butcher's broom and skullcap.

Sore/Strep Throat

Swollen Glands/Laryngitis/Hoarseness

The difference between a strep throat and a sore throat irritation from a cold is the onset of strep is rapid; a cold is slow. The throat is very sore with strep; not so with sore with a cold. There is a fever and aches with strep; mild achiness with a cold. There are swollen tender lymph nodes with strep throat; not with a cold. There are usually complications with strep, like streptococcal pneumonia or middle ear infection; sinusitis with a cold. Antibiotics work for strep throat; not usually for a cold, as it is viral not bacterial.

Hoarseness is the result of inflammation of the vocal chords and is typically the result of a virus or extensive yelling. Laryngitis, raspy, breathy voice, is often due to voice fatigue from a cold.

Common symptoms are sore aching inflamed throat and tonsils, swollen throat tissues, and difficulty talking.

Laryngitis is the inability to speak above a whisper because of swollen throat tissues.

Common symptoms are a viral or strep infection (if chronic it may be mononucleosis), tonsillitis, beginning of a cold or flu, consequences of smoking, lack of sleep, too many mucous forming foods, adrenal exhaustion, and stress.

Diet

Go on a short twenty-four-hour liquid cleansing diet or a three-day mucous cleaning diet. Drink citrus juices throughout the day. Use lemon juice and honey in water and drink potassium broth daily. Eat mainly fresh foods during healing. Have plenty of leafy green vegetables. Drink organic gourmet nutritional yeast or miso broth before retiring for the night.

Gargles: lemon juice and black tea with a pinch of cayenne, lemon juice, and sea salt in water, Golden Seal/Myrrh solution, Fenugreek/honey in water, Liquid Chlorophyll, (one half teaspoon in water), Myrrh tincture one half teaspoon in water, sage tea, or white oak bark tea. These are all effective gargle solutions for laryngitis and hoarseness caused by a sore or strep throat.

Allergies

Seasonal Hay-fever is caused by seasonal conditions such as dust, pollen or spores. This type of allergic reaction often occurs when the body has an excess accumulation of mucus, which harbors environmental irritants.

Respiratory Allergies result from two main areas environmental pollutants or chemical such as asbestos and smoke fumes.

Symptoms that occur are a runny nose and water-itchy eyes, sneezing and coughing attacks, irritated throat, chronic lung bronchial and sinus infections, skin itching and rashes, asthma, and headaches.

Common Causes are body sensitivity to pollen, spores, mold, and other airborne allergens that cause reaction.

Diet to help symptoms of allergies:

Go on a short 3 to 7-day liquid diet. Each day, have a glass of fresh carrot juice, potassium broth, cup of miso soup, and drink only bottled water. Then eat organically grown foods as much as possible. Avoid canned foods. Avoid caffeine and food sprayed with colorants and waxes. Have a bowl of high fiber cereal every morning. Eat legumes and sea vegetables and lots of green foods. Drink Aloe Gold juice and green tea. Use fiber and herbs colon cleanse, garlic oil, nettle caps, kelp, and iodine.

Tooth Ache

Wisdom tooth inflammation/Temporomandibular Joint Syndrome (TMJ)

Many dentists now realize that you need to see a nutritionist along with a dentist if you have chronic toothaches and infection. Diet, nutrition and lifestyle changes are indicated, not just more brushing and flossing. Natural healing wisdom about wisdom teeth, check to see that they're growing in straight, eat right, so they don't decay. Clean them well so you can keep them.

Common symptoms: Sore jaw or gums, dull or shooting pains, tooth or root nerve pain from cavity, tooth and jaw crowding from wisdom teeth coming in too big, misaligned, bleeding gums, TMJ symptoms.

Common causes: TMJ, poor bite, frequent clenching of the teeth, grinding at night.

Diet

Eat lots of crunch crisp food, to prevent recurring tooth problems. Eat celery, raw vegetables, nuts, and seeds, whole grain crackers, calcium rich foods; greens and go light on acid citrus' juices. Avoid soft gooey foods, no sweets, soft drinks or sodas.

For pain ice the jaw, poultice of Kava Kava caps, wild lettuce, cayenne, ginger, garlic, Echinacea, and myrrh extract drops. It can be used as a tea as well.

Constipation/Waste Management/ Colon/Bowel Health

The colon and bowel are the depository for all waste material after food nutrients have been extracted and processed to the blood stream. It is hardly any wonder that up to 90% of all diseases generate from an unclean colon. Decaying food ferments from gases as well as second and third generation toxins and the colon become a breeding ground for putrefactive bacteria, viruses, parasites, yeasts, and molds etc.

Common symptoms include infrequent bowl movements, flatulence and gas, fatigue, nausea and depression, nervousness, coated tongue, headaches, bad breath, and body odor.

Common causes of constipation are poor diets, too little fiber, too much fast food, fried, sugar, low residue foods, cheese, cow's milk, drugs, dairy, caffeine, alcohol, eating late at night, and lack of exercise.

Diet

Start with a short colon cleansing juice diet to rid the bowl of waste. Drink eight glasses of water every day. Follow a low fat, largely vegetarian diet, plenty of fruits, whole grains, salad greens, and cultured foods like yogurt. Make fiber the key food. Avoid all high fat foods. Drink aloe juice, dandelion extract tea, and senna tea, about four cups daily. Take bee pollen, omega 3 flax seed, fennel, and ginger.

Tonsillitis

Tonsil Lymph Inflammation

The tonsils are part of the lymphatic gland tissue on either side of the entrance to the throat. Their normal activity is straining and processing poison from the body. While the infection itself may not be serious, it always indicates a deeper immune response problem and can lead to serious problems such as rheumatic fever and nephritis scar tissues accumulates with every tonsillitis attack.

Common symptoms include swollen tonsils and lymph glands, difficulty swallowing, fever and tender throat, aches and pains in the back and extremities, bad breath because of the infection, ear infection, and hearing difficulty.

Common causes are a strep infection, poor diet that aggravates a sporadic infection with too many starches, sugar, dairy foods (pasteurized) not enough green vegetables, and soluble fiber foods, toxic build up, food allergies, and poor digestion.

Diet

Go on a three-day liquid cleansing diet to clear out body toxins. Eat only fresh foods for a week after the first three days. Drink lemon juice and water every morning. Drink plenty of high vitamin "C" juice. Have an onion and garlic broth each day.

Avoid sugars, pasteurized dairy products, and all junk foods. Drink six to eight glasses of bottled or purified water daily. Keep the body flushed. Drink aloe juice, ginger juice, mullein tea, lobelia tea, and thyme tea. As a gargle use Echinacea extract, garlic oil, and black walnut extract directly on throat. *Healthy Healing p. 415*

Kidney

Kidney function is vital to health. The kidneys are largely responsible for the elimination of waste products from protein breakdown; such as urea and ammonia. If the movement of salt, proteins or other bio-chemicals goes awry, a whole range of health problems arises from water retention to major kidney failure and mineral loss. Concentrated protein wastes can cause chronic inflammation of the kidney filtering tissues (nephritis, which is a severe inflammation of the kidney) and can overload the blood stream with toxins causing uremia, which is a form of blood poisoning. Naturopaths emphasize the importance of simple, high quality water for kidney health. Dehydration is the most common stress on the kidneys. Body purification systems operate efficiently only if the volume of water flowing through them is sufficient to carry away wastes. Drink six to eight glasses of water or other cleansing fluids daily for kidney health.

The bladder and kidney do more than just removes waste. They are part of a complex process that maintains body fluid stability. Urinary controls are involved.

Bladder

The brain is the control center for hormones and receptors for the body which regulates the use of fluids in the body. The hormones and receptors register what the body needs in the way of fluids for distribution of waste; therefore, sometimes a very little salt and waste is eliminated and at other times a lot of salt and waste are eliminated.

There comes a time when the bladder and kidney need to be cleansed. A bladder and kidney cleanse is simple and usually works right away. A three-day cleanse can often clear out toxic infections. When suffering from chronic lower back pain, irritated urination, frequent unexplained chills, fever, or nausea, and fluid retention, this could be caused by inflammation of a kidney.

Day one: For a gentle natural kidney cleanser try drinking ten glasses of bottled or purified water each day. Avoid dietary irritants on the kidney such as coffee, alcohol, and excessive proteins. Herbal supplements provide excellent support for a kidney cleanse. Use as liquids for the best results. Take a liquid green supplement daily such as Green Essence or Sun Chlorella. Apply wet, hot compresses on the lower back to speed cleansing. A hot and cold sitz bath, altering hot and cold, the night before beginning the cleanse process is helpful.

Day two: start the day by drinking a tea made of the either oat straw, corn silk, or crystal star. Option two: drink a glass of water with one teaspoon of lemon juice, one teaspoon of acidophilus, three teaspoons of concentrated cranberry juice. Another option is to take two tablespoons of apple cider vinegar with one teaspoon of honey in a glass of water.

Breakfast: A glass of watermelon juice or a glass of cranberry juice with one fourth teaspoon of vitamin C crystals.

Mid-morning: One cup of watermelon seed tea, cranberry juice or a glass of organic apple juice with one fourth teaspoon high potency acidophilus complex powder. Take two teaspoons of Braggs liquid aminos.

Lunch: Drink a vegetable drink, sun chlorella or crystal star energy green water, carrot juice, one cup of beets, cucumber juice, every other day.

Midafternoon: Drink a cup of healing herbs such as parsley, corn silk, or crystal star.

Dinner: Drink carrot juice with one teaspoon of liquid chlorophyll. Drink another cup of cranberry juice with one fourth teaspoon vitamin C crystals added.

Before bed: Drink a glass of papaya or apple juice with one fourth teaspoon high potency acidophilus powder.

After the cleansing add sea vegetables, whole grains and vegetables proteins to the diet. Continue with a morning green drink and drink some frequently during the rest of the month.

Day three: Repeat Day two.

A Twenty-Four-Hour Cleanse

The "Beginning" is usually the hardest part of doing cleansing. A block of time has to be set aside, all ingredients for the diet has to be gathered, and set eating times and patterns are essential during the process of cleansing. This disrupts the lifestyle of everybody in the household.

A twenty-four-hour detox is a juice and herbal tea cleanse. This allows the continuation of normal activities. It is a healing program. Even though it's quick, without the depth of vegetable juices needed for a major or chronic problem, it often is enough. It is definitely better than no cleanse at all. It makes a difference in the speed of healing.

Start the night before with a green leafy salad to give the bowels a good sweeping. For best results in the detoxification, dry brush the body before going to bed to open the pores for cleansing eliminations. The next twenty-four hours drink fresh juices and pure water. Upon waking, drink a glass of water with two fresh squeezed lemons and one table spoon of maple syrup. Take long walks during the day.

Mid-morning: Drink a glass of cranberry juice from concentrate.

Lunch: Drink a glass of fresh apple juice or apple/alfalfa sprouts juice with a packet of chlorella or green foods, green magma granules.

Midafternoon: Drink a cup of crystal star cleansing and purifying tea.

Dinner: Drink a glass of papaya/pineapple juice to enhance enzyme production or drink a glass of apple juice with one packet of sun chlorella or green foods green magna granules.

Before bed: Drink a cup of mint tea or a cup of hot water with one teaspoon of organic gourmet's nutritional yeast extract or a cup miso soup for relaxation and strength for the next day.

The next morning: Break the fast by eating fresh fruits and yogurt. Eat light at the beginning with raw foods during the day and have a simple prepared low-fat dinner in the evening.

Before bed: bathe in seaweed or mineral enhanced water. Get a full eight hours of rest. Start the next morning as the first day of a healthy diet change aimed at restoring health.

The Wonderful Heart

The great throbbing center of all human life and activity is the heart. No other organ carries so much responsibility for the rest of the body. Every part of the human system is entirely dependent upon heart. The lungs enable us to breathe while the kidney filters out the waste material from the blood. The one great organ upon which all others depend is the heart. Day and night the heart constantly beats. While one is resting it beats quietly and slowly, conserving its great powers for the time when they might be sorely needed. If an emergency should arise, the heart will immediately quicken its pace, speeding up the circulation of blood wherever it may be needed.

Keep the Heart Healthy

When the heart is strong and healthy, the whole-body benefits. When it is sick, the whole body suffers. That is why it is important to take care of the heart. On the condition of the heart all life depends, in order to get the very best out of life. A heart that has been damaged can be strained beyond its limits.

Common symptoms are irregular or rapid heartbeat, uncomfortable awareness of your heartbeat, skipped heartbeats, and shortness of breath, a feeling that you cannot breathe, light-headedness, and often chest discomfort.

Common causes are a poor diet, too much refined sugar, saturated fats, lack of exercise, obesity, smoking, stressful lifestyle, high blood pressure, and diabetes.

Diet

Keep the diet low in fats, salt, and calories. Have a fresh green salad daily. Have whole grains and protein every day. Add sunflower and sesame seeds, miso soup, rice and oat brain, and green leafy vegetables to the diet. Take green drink once a week. Helpful teas, cayenne, ginger caps, hawthorn, ginseng, butcher's broom, peppermint and sage.

Diabetes

Most humans are able to live fairly normal lives when not limited by any serious handicaps. Follow regular routines of eating, sleeping, working, and recreation. To the majority of people, it matters little if they miss a meal now and then. Some people are not so fortunate. They may appear normal in every way. They may run into certain problems when it comes to eating. They may actually become ill when they miss a meal, others become cold and clammy all over. They feel as if they are drained of all energy. Their muscles refuse to work properly. They are not able to adjust to certain chemical changes. They may seem to be weak. The truth is, they may have diabetes mellitus. Such a person may not be fully aware of their true condition. They may eat large amounts of food while still losing weight or on the other hand, gaining rapidly. He or she owes it to themselves to have a complete medical examination. This person might have diabetes or some other condition affecting the endocrine glands.

What is Diabetes?

Diabetes is a strange disease; no one knows its true cause. Some of the trouble seems to arise in the tail of the pancreas where the small island of Langerhans cells are located. These little glands produce a powerful hormone that aids the body in storing nutriment instead of allowing it to drain away in the urine. This hormone is called insulin.

Some people are unable to produce enough insulin to meet their own needs. As a result, their blood sugar rises to a very high level and excess glucose spills over into the urine.

If this continues for a long enough time, the person may find himself becoming weaker. Unless he is properly treated, he may become ill and die. The pancreas is not the only organ concerned with this strange disease; the liver and the thyroid all seem to play some part. Keeping the blood sugar at a more or less constant level is a complex process requiring the normal function of all the endocrine glands. When the pancreas does not produce enough insulin, the other glands are out of balance and the blood sugar level rises. All these reactions depend on the presence of insulin, a hormone that is essential for growth and life itself. Diabetes has been known for thousands of years but only about two hundred years ago doctors found that diabetic patients were losing large quantities of sugar in their urine.

Danger Signals of Diabetes

Extreme thirst, loss of weight, large quantities of urine, chronic skin trouble, cuts and bruises heal slowly if at all. In children; vomit, lapse into coma, a high blood sugar, Diabetic Acidosis, too little insulin or else too much food. (A type of pain)

Serious Complications

The body needs food. The body is a living engine. It needs food to keep it going. The body stores food as carbohydrates and fats to use when needed. The body's preference is sugar and carbohydrates but when not available will use fats. Ketones are chemicals the liver makes. One produces them when there is not enough insulin in the body to turn sugar (or glucose) into energy. A person needs another source, so the body uses fat instead. The liver turns this fat into ketones, a type of acid, and sends them to the bloodstream. Pregnant women, having an overactive thyroid gland, being obese/overweight; all with such conditions run a risk of serious complications as these conditions puts a strain on the pancreas. Arteriosclerosis and ulcers; hardening of the arteries occur more frequently.

Other serious changes; eyes change retinitis is a serious occurrence and common in patients. Another eye problem is cataracts in older people who have had diabetes for five years or longer.

Urinary problems: Kidney infections of the urinary tract; the most serious complication involving the kidney is the Kimmelstiel-Wilson syndrome and the kidneys are damaged. It affects the network of tiny blood vessels (the microvascular) in the glomerulus, a key structure in the kidney that is composed of capillary blood vessels and which is critically necessary for the filtration of the blood. He loses albumin in the urine, which is a protein made by the liver. Albumin helps keep fluid in the bloodstream so it doesn't leak into other tissues. In addition, he suffers from high blood pressure and swelling as edema in parts of his body.

Acidosis is a very serious complication. Renal tubular acidosis occurs when the kidneys are unable to excrete acids into the urine. Fifty percent of all diabetics who died suffered from complications due to acidosis and coma. Acidosis or acid poisoning may occur with any infection whether in the digestive tract, urinary organs, or the skin.

Making the Diagnosis

Diabetes is one condition that is readily recognized today. The first step is to have a urine test and have a blood sugar test. Normal fasting blood sugar is usually 80 and 120 mg per 100 mil.

Part Six:

Instruction on Eating

Most of the diseases and suffering are mainly due because of error in diet. The major portion of the diet should consist of fruits and vegetables, prepared in a natural tasty way. Vary the diet but do not eat too many varieties at one meal. Make your meals simple. Use whole grains, wheat, brown rice, and discard the use of refined grains such as white flour and white rice. Eliminate rich concentrated foods containing sugar, fats, and oils. Use low salt and little or no meat from animals.

Eat at the same time each day. The stomach functions best on a regular schedule. Allow four to five hours from the end of each meal before beginning the next meal. Do not eat between meals. This causes the partially digested food in the stomach to spoil and ferment. Breakfast should be the largest meal of the day. If supper is eaten, it should be small and at least two to three hours before bedtime. Eat enough to maintain health but do not overeat. Too much food dulls the mind, causes fatigue, increased diseases, and shortens life.

Eat food slowly; chew the food thoroughly to increase the enjoyment and the nutritional benefits of it. Meal time should not be hurried, enjoy your meal. Drink enough water daily to keep the urine pale. Drink liquids between meals. Drinking water or any other liquid during meals delays digestion. Stagnation of food in the stomach is one of the causes of ulcers and gastritis.

Stomach Irritants

The following are irritants to the stomach: All hot chili peppers, spices such as ginger, cinnamon, and nutmeg, alcoholic beverages and foods having a fermenting, putrefying or rotting phase in processing, such as sauerkraut, cheese, soy sauce, and vinegar found in pickles, mayonnaise, catsup, mustard, and salad dressings. Caffeine found in coffee, tea, and colas, theobromine (chocolate) and the use of tobacco, milk, eggs, and sugar combinations, baking soda and baking powder, unripe or over-ripe fruit are stomach irritants. Fruits and vegetables eaten at the same time, foods too hot or too cold, meals less than five hours apart, eating too much, eating too fast, eating too late at night. All of these are stomach irritants.

Exercise

Exercise is an absolute requirement for body strength and development. More people die from lack of exercise than too much. Daily exercise is beneficial for people of all ages. Exercise promotes a sense of well-being and prevents disease; it also aids in the recovery from disease. "If those who are sick would exercise their muscles daily in outdoor work, using brain and muscle properly, weakness and languor would disappear." Health would take the place of disease and strength would take the place of feebleness. *(Medical Ministry p. 297).*

He giveth power to the faint; and to them that have no might He increaseth strength. Even the youths shall faint and be weary, and the young men shall utterly fall: But they that wait upon the LORD shall mount up with wings as eagles; they shall run, and not be weary; and they shall walk, and not faint. *Isaiah 40:29-31.*

The best exercise is walking in the invigorating morning air of heaven. Gardening and outside work will bring health and strength to move and health of muscles; cultivating flowers, fruits, and vegetables is necessary for healthful circulation of the blood. It also helps the brain, lungs, and inflammation of the liver. Exercise must be regular. Exercise regulates the blood pressure. Exercise slows down the aging process. Exercise aids digestion (briskly walk after meals). Exercise helps to regulate the body's weight. Exercise strengthens the immune system. Exercise reduces stress. Exercise lifts gloom from the mind. Exercise improves clean thinking. Exercise prevents coronary heart disease, hypertension, obesity, osteoporosis, and diabetes. Exercise improves sleep and mental outlook on life.

Water

Man can live up to six weeks without food but only a few days without water. A continuous supply of water is needed for all living things. Every cell of the body needs water. Water makes up about 60% of our total body weight. The Bible tells how to satisfy the thirst. "If any man thirst, let him come unto Me, and drink." John 7:37 last part. In health and in sickness, pure water is one of heaven's choicest blessings. It is the beverage which God provided to quench the thirst of animals and man.

The body's organs and tissues require large quantities of water in order to work effectively. Water keeps the body temperature within a normal range. The evaporation of perspiration on the skin's surface helps bring down fever. Water produces the fluid that constantly moistens the eyes. Without tears, the eyes would become dry and inflamed resulting in loss of sight. Water is needed to lubricate and cushion the bones and joints. Water is necessary for the production of saliva and digestives juices. Water relieves both physical and mental fatigue. The brain is approximately 85% water. It is surprising that drinking one glass of water (eight ounces) every ten minutes for one hour relieves many headaches. Fortunately, the body has wonderful ways to conserve its water. Approximately ten glasses of water are eliminated daily through the following ways: kidneys excrete five and one half glasses through urine, the skin two glasses through perspiration, the lungs loose two glasses through the breath, and the gastrointestinal tract uses one half glass in the stool.

The body receives a daily supply of water from the intake of food, three glasses, and from the metabolic processes, one and a half glass. One must drink six or more glasses of water to replace the body's average daily water losses. There are some conditions that increase the body's water loss. Some of those conditions are: high fever, hard physical work, other activity that increases sweating, illnesses such as common cold that increases upper respiratory tract secretions, dry air or hot air or very cold winter air; vomiting and diarrhea, nursing mother, high protein foods, high salt or sugar intake, vitamin/mineral supplements for the kidney to remove waste. Recommendation for water intake: drink two glasses upon rising, two glasses mid-morning, two glasses mid-afternoon, and two glasses before bedtime.

The body requires water for breathing, digestion, elimination, hormone secretion, lubrication of muscles, bones, tendons, protection from injury by cushioning tissues, personal hygiene, water treatments, cleanliness of home and clothes. *(1905 Ministry of Healing p. 419, Letter 35 1809).*

Sunlight

The sunshine helps produce Vitamin D. All would become ill without it. "Truly the light is sweet, and a pleasant thing it is for the eyes to behold the sun." *Ecclesiastes 11:7* It is one of nature's most powerful healing agents. Sunlight improves the circulation of the blood. It increases the cardiac output, the amount of blood that is pumped by the heart. Sunlight increases the amount of oxygen carried through the blood. It helps to regulate the blood pressure towards a normal healthy level. It increases the number of white blood cells and stimulates their ability to destroy both germs and cancer cells, increases gamma globulin – a protein that helps the body fight infection. It is an effective treatment for jaundice in newborn infants, improves liver function, helps the body to eliminate toxins, and help to lower the blood sugar that is too high (in diabetes). Sunlight may decrease cholesterol by more than 30%, increases the body metabolism by stimulating thyroid gland function, promote healing.

"In the building of houses, it is especially important to secure thorough ventilation and plenty of sunlight. Let there be a current of air and an abundance of light in every room in the house. Sleeping rooms should be so arranged as to have a free circulation of air day and night. No room is fit to be occupied as a sleeping room unless it can be thrown open daily to the air and sunshine." *Ministry of Healing 274* "But unto you that fear My name shall the Sun of Righteousness arise with healing in His wings." *Malachi 4:2 first part.*

Temperance

Intemperance lies at the foundation of all the evil in our world. *Temperance p. 165* A temperate appetite cleans the mind to perfect Christian character for God's glory and service. Whether therefore ye eat, or drink, or whatsoever ye do, do all to the glory of God. *1 Corinthians 10:31.*

By practicing temperance in eating, in drinking, in dressing, in labor, and in all things, we can do for ourselves what no physician can for us. *(My Life Today p. 142).*

The controlling power of appetite will prove the ruin of thousands, when, if they had conquered on this point, they would have had moral power to gain the victory over every other temptation of Satan. But those who are slaves to appetite will fail in perfecting Christian character. *(Counsels on Diet and Foods p. 59).*

There is no place in the Bible where it sanctions the use of intoxicating wines. Proverbs put it this way: "Wine is a mocker, strong drink is raging: and whosoever is deceived thereby is not wise." Proverbs 20:1. The wine that Christ made from water at the marriage feast of Cana was the pure juice of the grape. This is the 'new wine... found in the cluster,' of which the Scriptures say, 'Destroy it not; for a blessing is in it.' Isaiah 65:8. This is clearly speaking about grapes on the vine (the fruit of the vine) before it is processed not to be destroyed. *(Ministry of Healing p. 333).*

Tea and coffee drinking is a sin, an injurious indulgence, which, like other evils, injures the soul. These darling idols create an excitement, a morbid action of the nervous system; and after immediate influence of the stimulants is gone, it lets down below par just to that degree that its stimulating properties elevated above par. *(Counsels on Diet and Foods p. 425).*

Alcoholism is a leading cause of disease and death. It poisons every tissue of the body, the brain, nervous system, the heart, liver, gastrointestinal tract, the immune system, and causes the red blood cells to clump together, slowing the circulation of the red blood cells throughout the body.

Tobacco is a legal product, if used, it could cause death. Smoking injures every tissue of the body. Some of the poisons found in cigarettes, which causes cancer are: nicotine, carbon monoxide, cyanide, and tar.

Dress

The Bible teaches modesty in dress. "In like manner also, that women adorn themselves in modest apparel, with shamefacedness and sobriety; not with braided hair, or gold, or pearls, or costly array." 1 Timothy 2:10. The most beautiful dress He (Christ) bids us wear: "Whose adorning let it not be that outward adorning of plaiting the hair, and of wearing of gold or of putting of apparel; But let it be the hidden man of the heart, in that which is not corruptible, even the ornament of a meek and quiet spirit, which is in the sight in God of great price." 1 Peter 3:3-4.

It is an easy matter to lose the health, but it is difficult to regain it.... We cannot afford to dwarf or cripple a single function of the mind or body by overwork or abuse of any part of the living machinery. *(My Life Today p. 142).*

Fresh Air

Fresh air promotes a healthful circulation of the blood. It refreshes and strengthens the body. Pure air soothes the nerves, excites the appetite, and helps the food to digest. "The breath of the Almighty hath given me life." Job 33:4 last part.

Fresh air gives the mind composure and serenity. Man might live five to six weeks without food, only a few days without water, but only a few minutes without air. The lungs inflate with breathing more than 600 million times during an average lifetime. No matter where we live, in the cold, the desert, in the city smog and pollution, or in the hot steamy jungle, air. The air sacs or the alveoli deep in the lungs need air that is warm, moist, and free of dust, smoke and germs. The Alveoli are tiny air sacs in your lungs that take up the oxygen you breathe in and keep your body going. Although they're microscopic, alveoli are the workhorses of your respiratory system. You have about 480 million alveoli, located at the end of bronchial tubes. When you breathe in, the alveoli expand to take in oxygen. When you breathe out, the alveoli shrink to expel carbon dioxide.... The oxygen you breathe in diffuses through the alveoli and the capillaries into the blood. The carbon dioxide you breathe out is diffused from the capillaries to the alveoli, up the bronchial tree and out your mouth. Medically reviewed by Suzanne Falck, MD on November 26, 2018–Written by Marjorie Hecht. The lungs receive this precious cargo through the nasal passages. The lungs and the nasal passages are continually exposed to respiratory pathogens, toxins, and particulate matter.

The nasal passages condition the air inhaled through the nose. In cold weather, the nasal blood vessels widen or dilate, heating the incoming air. In hot weather, the blood vessels shrink, helping to cool the incoming air. Air passes into the bronchial airway that is lined with tiny hair-like cilia. Cilia are complex structures of paranasal sinus mucosa in which its function is critical to respiratory defense. Good posture deep breathing exercises facilitate the flow of pure air deep into the lungs. Reading aloud, singing, climbing stairs or hills can increase the efficiency of the lungs. For best health, live in the country rather than the city. "From the standpoint of health, the smoke and dust of the cities are very objectionable... Sometimes an invalid is poisoned by his own breath." *(Testimony Volume 7, p. 82).*

Rest

The Bible gives the source of spiritual rest. "Come unto Me, all ye that labor and are heavy laden, and I will give you rest. Take My yoke upon you and learn of Me; for I am meek and lowly in heart: and ye shall find rest unto your souls." Matthew 11:28-29 Rest is absolutely essential to both physical and mental health. Sometime a change in the type of work may benefit one's health. For example, a change from mental to physical labor will benefit. Nearly one third of life is spent in sleep. During sleep both the body's physical and mental functions are restored. The best quality of sleep is during the hours before midnight. Bedtime should be no later than 10:00 p.m. We sleep best if our stomach can also rest from its work of digestion at least three hours after eating before retiring for the night. Problems result from insufficient sleep; irritability, memory loss, depression and difficulty concentrating all stems from the lack of sleep. Lack of sleep promotes disease, by diminishing the body's ability to restore and repair its tissues and organs. Rest versus peace: "Peace I leave with you, My peace I give unto you: not as the world giveth, give I unto you." John 14:27 first part. "Many of the diseases from which men suffer are the result of mental depression. Grief, anxiety, discontent, remorse, guilt, distrust, all tend to break down the life forces and to invite decay and death." *(Ministry of Healing p. 241).*

The Sabbath was created as a special day of rest. A time for God's people to receive physical, mental, and spiritual restoration as a blessing from Him. "And God did rest the seventh day from all His works." Hebrews 4:4 last part.

Trust in Divine Power

In order to have perfect health, our hearts must be filled with love and hope and joy in the Lord. We should cooperate with God in the care of our bodies. The very best physical, mental and spiritual health possible is attained only by connecting with the power of God. Faith and trust connecting with divine power undergirds all other health laws. Love for God is essential for life and health. The better the total health, the greater will be the ability to honor and glorify the Creator. Most people may follow the ten laws perfect, but perfect health is possible only by including the eight health laws.

God is the Author of all law. These laws include the Moral Law or the Ten Commandments, Civil Law, (without which Nations cannot exist), Natural Law (of nature), Man's Being (all functions of human body), Physical (including the entire man, mental and moral). Jesus lived in perfect obedience to His heavenly Father's will in all laws. "For I came down from heaven, not to do mine own will, but the will of Him that sent Me." John 6:38. Christ's followers are to imitate His example. "If ye love Me, keep My commandments." John 14:15. The Bible teaches how mankind is to relate to Heaven's Laws. If ye love Me, keep (obey) My commandments. It is not only the privilege, but the sacred duty of man. Heaven's perfect health is achieved through our connection with God, our cooperation with heaven's laws, our service to God, our service for others, and our relationship with God.

As Christians equipped for battle, one must put on the whole armor of God. Be prepared to meet His spiritual enemies with the weapons that God has provided us. Remember David? Saul's armor did not fit David and Goliath's armor was useless against David's stone. A stray arrow found a crack in Ahab's armor. This is why humanity must put on the unfailing armor of God. Notice carefully and wear it to live victoriously.

First is the garment of truth. Next the breastplate of righteousness, then the shoes of peace, the shield of faith, the helmet of salvation, and the sword of the Spirit, which is the word of God. Wear the whole armor of God, "that ye may be able to stand against the wiles of the devil." Ephesians 6:11

last part. "Wherefore take unto you the whole armor of God, that ye may be able to withstand in the evil day, and having done all, to stand." Verse 13.

The Sword: A soldier traveling in enemy territory never let his sword out of his reach. A Christian should "be ready always to give an answer to every man that asketh you a reason of the hope that is in you with meekness and fear:" 1 Peter 3:15 last part. Apostle Paul, often threatened with danger, beaten, stoned, and mobbed, shipwrecked and imprisoned, could say, "thanks be unto God, which always causeth us to triumph in Christ..."
2 Corinthians 2:14.

Belt of Truth: The girdle or belt about the waist held together the soldier's garments which might otherwise hindered his movements while engaging in battle. The significance here is God does not want one to simply look at the truth. He wants people to wear it, wrapped around not only does the belt hold everything in place, it also secures a place to carry the sheath that holds the sword of the Spirit. The belt of truth also means wearing Christ. He is the way, the truth and the life. John 14:6. As many who have been baptized into Christ has put on Christ. Galatians 3:27.

Breastplate of Righteousness: In the Bible, the breastplate was an article of important defense that protected the front of the vital organs from mortal wounds. It was often composed of a solid piece of metal. It could also contain small pieces that were sewed to cloth or leather that overlapped like the scales of a fish. They could number as many as seven hundred to one thousand per coat. When the sun shone direct on the armor, it could burn or become very hot. To avoid being burnt or pinched by moving metal plates, the soldiers always wore a robe under the armor. In other words, the breastplate of righteousness is always in partnership with the robe of Jesus Righteousness. Job 29:14 says: "I put on righteousness, and it clothed me": Keep in mind the High Priest wore a golden breastplate over his linen robe, with the names of the twelve tribes of Israel on it. "And Aaron shall bear the names of the children of Israel in the breastplate of judgment upon his heart, when he goeth in unto the holy place, for a memorial before the LORD continually." Exodus 28:29. Another interesting aspect of the breastplate was that it offered no protection to the persons' back. It was assumed that soldiers would not turn their back toward the enemy to retreat.

Likewise, Christian soldiers should stand firm and never surrender any ground to the devil. Let the devil flee. "Submit yourself therefore to God. Resist the devil, and he will flee from you." James 4:10.

Shield of Faith: The shield was usually made of wood or bronze. The shield was the warrior's first line of defense. It was big enough to protect the whole body. The shield was firmly strapped to the soldier's hand and forearm so he could resist the mighty blows of the enemy's sword without fear of dropping. When the soldiers crouch down under a hail of arrows, having faith in Christ's blood is our first defense against the great accuser. The devil is constantly firing volley after volley of those flaming arrows. The purpose of this shield of faith is to deflect the fiery darts of the enemy and prevent them from ever making contact. Many Christians fall on the battlefield and fail to overcome evil because they wait until they are immersed in the fire of temptation before making any effort to resist. At that point, it is often too late. Hold up the shield of faith and do all in power to keep as much distance as possible. There is no time to lose. God is faithful, "who will not suffer you to be tempted above that ye are able; but will with the temptation also make a way to escape, that ye may be able to bear it." 1 Corinthians 10:13 last part.

Helmet of Salvation: Several stories in the Bible stress the importance of protecting the head. King Abimelech died because he charged a city wall without putting on his helmet. A woman cast a piece of millstone upon his head to brake his skull. Judges 9:55. Wearing a helmet improperly proved to be a fatal mistake. Goliath became outraged that David would dare come against him with nothing but a shepherd's staff and a sling in his hand. Goliath carelessly pushed back his helmet. Minutes later a smooth stone sunk deep into his forehead. 1 Samuel 17:40-49. The helmet of salvation does not only keep out the rocks but it also keeps in the brains. The mind should not be open to any and everything. As one studies God's word, there should be a settling into the truth, "That we henceforth be no more children, tossed to and fro, and carried about with every wind of doctrine," Ephesians 4:14 first part. Only in eternity will we appreciate them. Keep the helmet in place and guard these avenues to the soul, nostrils, ears, eyes, and the mouth from the neck up.

Shoes of Gospel: "How beautiful upon the mountains are the feet of him that bringeth good tidings, that publisheth peace; that bringeth good tidings of good, that publisheth salvation" Isaiah 52:7 first part. The foot in Bible symbol "the walk" or the direction of one's walk in their personal life. Having their feet shod with the preparation of the gospel, having a good footing to prevent backsliding. Having good footing gives victory over sins and the enemy. Never remove your gospel shoes and God will be with you always. Your sandals will never ware out. Deuteronomy 29:5. Remember the children of Israel?

Sword of the Word: "For the Word of God is quick, and powerful, and sharper than any two-edged sword, piercing even to the dividing asunder of soul and spirit, and of the joints and marrow, and is a discerner of the thoughts and intents of the heart." Hebrews 4:12. The word of God has a dividing effect. The two edges of the Spirit's sword are the two witnesses of God's word, the Old and New Testaments. We must be ready to apply the sword to our lives. "But sanctify the Lord God in your hearts: and be ready always to give an answer to every man that asketh you a reason of the hope that is in you with meekness and fear:" 1 Peter 3:15

Always with Prayer: The most important piece of armament is prayer. Every general knows that victory depends on the army with the strongest elements. In the warfare, the strongest element is watchfulness and prayer. "Watch and pray, that ye enter not into temptation: the spirit indeed is willing, but the flesh is weak." Matthew 26:41 Gideon's soldiers were chosen based upon their watchfulness. They caught the enemy sleeping and won the battle. The best armor is useless if the soldiers are found sleeping. People are commanded to watch and pray. Prayer is the link that connects one with Christ. It is said at times prayer is the key that opens heaven's store house. "Every sincere prayer is heard in heaven. It may not be fluently expressed; but if the heart is in it, it will ascend to the sanctuary where

Jesus ministers, and He will present it to the Father without one awkward, stammering word, beautiful and fragrant with the incense of His own perfection. *Desire of Ages, p. 667.* There should be a hatred of sin. God hears prayer when the sinner is ready to exchange sin for righteousness. "But to pray in Christ's name means much. It means that we are to accept His character, manifest His spirit, and work His works. The Savior's promise is given on condition. "If ye love Me, He says, "keep My commandments." He saves men, not in sin, but from sin; and those who love Him will show their love by obedience." *Desire of Ages, p. 668.* Be sober, be vigilant; because your adversary the devil, as a roaring lion, walketh about seeking whom he may devour" 1 Peter 5:8. Prayer is most essential. We are admonished to "Pray without ceasing" 1 Thessalonians 5:17. As God's soldiers, it is time to stop simply having the word, the Bible, but to begin obeying. Fight the good fight of faith.

You May Have Power

It is written how the battle will end, and who will have the final victory. The One who gives the armor guarantees, with this promise, "And the gates of hell shall not prevail against it." Matthew 15:18 last part. Peter admonishes that have the power for victory because Jesus gave it. He said "According as

His divine power hath given unto all things that pertain unto life and godliness, through the knowledge of him that hath called all to glory and virtue:" 2 Peter 1:3. Our Savior further told us in John 15:5 "for without me ye can do nothing." Last part. We also have this assurance, "I can do all things through Christ which strengthened me" Philippians 4:13. All that is needed was purchased at Calvary with the blood of Christ, the Son of God. "God so loved the world that He gave." John 3:16 first part.

Just as Jonathan so loved David that he gave him his armor, his sword, robe, yes, his bow and girdle, 1 Samuel 18:3-4. Jesus Christ called this powerful invisible force that He gives the Holy Spirit. He told His disciples to pray for it in John 14:26 "But the Comforter, which is the Holy Ghost, whom the Father will send in my name, He shall teach you all things, and bring all things to your remembrance, whatsoever I have said unto you." Jesus told His disciples that it was to their advantage that He go away, "Nevertheless I tell you the truth; it is expedient for you that I go away: for if I go not away, the Comforter will not come unto you; but if I depart, I will send Him unto you." John 16:7. He said the Holy Spirit whom the Father will send will teach you all things and bring to remembrance all He said.

After His resurrection, He recalled these things to their mind. In Luke 24:44 "And he said unto them, These are the words which I spake unto you, while I was yet with you, that all things must be fulfilled, which were written in the law of Moses, and in the prophets, and in the psalms, concerning me." He told them in Acts 1:8 "But ye shall receive power, after that the Holy Ghost is come upon you:" first part. The power of the Holy Spirit was not confined to healing, it was active in every activity of the Church. This power is available today. Ephesians 4:13 "Till we all come in the unity of the faith, and of the knowledge of the Son of God, unto a perfect man, unto the measure of the stature of the fulness of Christ:" God uses the Holy Spirit to change man's hearts and lives.

Part Seven:

Let Food Be Your Medicine and Medicine Be Your Food

Many who violate the laws of health are ignorant of the law of living, eating, drinking, and working for health. They then become sick with some kind of illness. They do not realize that their condition is caused by violating the laws of nature and health. They have been neglecting proper diet, the use of pure water, fresh air, sunshine, rest, and nature's remedies. Nature would restore the body to its original health. There is a wonderful science in nature's trees, herbs, roots, and flowers, which man has never yet fathomed.

God has provided a remedy for every disease that might affect people. The Creator foresaw the wretched condition of mankind in these days, and made provision in nature for all the ills of man. If they would make use of only these remedies that God has given for the service of man, it would bring an untold blessing to the world. The most important subject should be: How can we live our allotted time without suffering? God has surely made this possible.

The Creator of the universe made man out of the ground. The different properties which are found in the earth are found in man. The fruits, grains, nuts, and vegetables contain the same elements which are in the earth. "My people are destroyed for lack of knowledge:" Hosea 4:6 first part, is surely being fulfilled. "And by the river upon the bank thereof, on this side and on that side, shall grow all trees for meat, whose leaf shall not fade, neither shall the fruit thereof be consumed: it shall bring forth new fruit according to his months, because their waters they issued out of the sanctuary: and the fruit thereof shall be for meat, and the leaf thereof for medicine." Ezekiel 47:12. There are wonderful life-giving properties in fruit, if eaten properly.

Fruit Diet

All fruits contain acid, which are necessary for proper elimination of toxins, poisonous acids, and other impurities. Natural acids are highly alkaline. Germs cannot grow and live in fruit juice. Fresh fruits are more effective citric, malic acids are most powerful.

Malic acid is an organic compound. It is dicarboxylic acid that is made of living organisms, contributes to the sour taste of fruits, and is used as a food additive. Malic acid is found in pineapple, apples, quinces, pears, apricots, plums, peaches, cherries, currants, goose-berry, strawberries, raspberries, elderberries, grapes, and tomatoes.

Tartaric acid is a white, crystalline organic acid that occurs naturally in many fruits, most notably in grapes, but also in bananas, tamarinds, avocados and citrus fruits. It is important in treating all diseases of hyper acidity such as lung diseases, sore throat, indigestion, etc.

Oxalic acid is an organic compound found in many plants. These include leafy greens, vegetables, fruits, and is especially good for constipation and inactive liver.

Lactic acid is found in fermented soybean and is good in treating hardening of the arteries.

Meat Eating

The argument that flesh must be eaten in order to supply the body sufficient protein is unreasonable; it is found in abundance in beans, peas, lentils, all kinds of nuts, and also some fruits. The nutritive value of meat broths is practically nothing. They contain uric acid and other poisons. Excessive uric acid causes rheumatism, Bright's disease, kidney stones, gout, gallstones, and headaches. Plants perfectly take the place of meat.

Pecans, filberts, English walnuts, almonds, hickory, chestnut (aka white walnut), are abundant in growth promoting vitamins. Nuts should not be used as a dainty: they should be staple articles for the diet. The popular ideal that nuts are hard to digest has no foundation. Eating nuts at the end of a meal, when in all probability more food of highly nutritious nature has been eaten than necessary, is very injurious. It is equally injurious to eat in between meals. Improper mastication is a common cause of indigestion from the use of nuts. Peanuts should be heated slightly to remove skin. Other nuts may be blanched and crushed without roasting. When nuts are over-roasted, it makes them very difficult to digest.

Nuts and Seeds

Name	**Amt**	**Cal**	**Protein**	**CHO**	**Fiber**
Almonds	1 oz	163	6.0g	6.1g	3.5g
Brazil	1 oz	186	4.1g	3.5g	2.1g
Cashew	1 oz	157	5.2g	8.6g	0.9g
Hazelnut	1 oz	178	4.2g	4.7g	2.7g
Macadamia	1 oz	204	2.2g	3.9g	2.4g
Pecan	1 oz	196	2.6g	3.9g	2.7g
Pistachio	1 oz	159	5.8g	7.8g	2.9g
Walnut	1 oz	185	4.3g	3.9g	1.9g

Beans and Legumes

Name	Amt	Cal	Protein	CHO	Fiber
Soybean/ Edamame	1 cup	296	31.3g	14.4g	10.3
Lentils	1 cup	230	17.9	39.9g	15.6g
Large White Beans	1 cup	249	17.4	44.9g	11.3g
Cranberry (Roman) Bean	1 cup	241	16.5g	43.3g	15.2g
Split Peas	1 cup	231	16.3g	41.4g	16.3g
Pinto Beans	1 cup	245	15.4g	44.8g	15.4g
Kidney Beans	1 cup	225	15.3g	40.4g	11.3g
Black Beans	1 cup	227	15.2g	40.8g	15g
Navy Beans	1 cup	255	15g	47.4g	19.1g
Lima Beans	1 cup	216	14.7g	39.3g	13.2g

Grains

Name	Amt	Cal	Protein	CHO	Fiber
Kamut (Wheat)	1 cup	227	9.8g	47.5g	7.4g
Teff	1 cup	255	9.8g	50g	7.1g
Quinoa	1 cup	222	8.1g	39.4g	5.2g
Whole Wheat Pasta	1 cup	174	7g	35.2g	4.6g
Wild Rice	1 cup	166	6.5g	35g	3g
Millet	1 cup	207	2.3g	41.2g	2.3g
Couscous	1 cup	176	6g	36.5g	2.2g
Oatmeal	1 cup	166	5.9g	28.1g	4g
Buckwheat	1 cup	155	5.7g	35.5g	4.5g
Cornmeal (Grits)	1 cup	182	4.4g	37.9g	2.1g

Vegetables

Name	Amt	Cal	Protein	CHO	Fiber
Soybean Sprouts	1 cup	85	9.2g	6.7g	0.8g
Green Peas (Cooked)	1 cup	134	8.6g	25g	8.8g
Spinach (Cooked)	1 cup	41	5.3g	6.8g	4.3g
Yellow Sweet Corn	1 cup	125	4.7g	27.1g	2.9g
Asparagus (Cooked)	1 cup	40	4.3g	7.4g	3.6g
Arti-chokes Globe or French	1 cup	60	4.2g	13.5g	6.9g
Brussels Sprouts (Cooked)	1 cup	56	4g	11.1g	4.1g
Mushrooms White (Cooked)	1 cup	28	3.9g	4.4g	1.9g
Broccoli (Cooked)	1 cup	55	3.7g	11.2g	5.1g

Fruit

Name	Amt	Cal	Protein	CHO	Fiber
Guavas	1 cup	112	4.2g	23.6g	8.9g
Avocado	1 cup	240	3.g	12.8g	10.1g
Apricot	1 cup halves	74	2.2g	17.2g	3.1g
Kiwi	1 cup sliced	110	2.1g	26.4g	5.4g
Blackberries	1 cup	62	2g	13.8g	7.6g
Oranges	1 cup sections	85	1.7g	21.2g	4.3g
Bananas	1 medium	105	1.3g	27g	3.1g
Cantaloupe	1 cup balls	60	1.5g	14.4g	1.6g
Raspberries	1 cup	64	1.5g	14.7g	8g
Peaches	1 cup slices	60	1.4g	14.7g	2.3g

All food protein values taken from *https://www.myfooddata.com.*

Common Salt

Salt should be used very sparingly. It contains chloride of sodium, which is an inorganic mineral, which cannot be used by any cell structure of the body. It irritates the stomach and blood stream. It is indigestible and hinders the digestion of other foods. It is one of the causes of rheumatism, dizziness, cancer, and scurfy by putting harmful minerals into the system. Sodium salts are plentifully found in fruits and vegetables, such as tomatoes, asparagus, celery, spinach, kale, radishes, turnips, carrots, lettuce, strawberries, and many others. When salt is omitted, a person soon enjoys the flavor of the food more. Salt must not be used when dropsy, hyperacidity, Bright's disease, gastric ulcer, obesity, and epilepsy are present.

Vital Nutrients

Carbohydrates supply energy. Cellulose is the framework of fruits and vegetables and supplies bulk, which aids in normal intestinal peristalsis and stimulates the bowels. Fats supply energy in a very concentrated form and are also foods. Mineral matter supplies building materials and helps regulate the body processes. Mineral salts are necessary for blood making and tissue building. Proteins supply energy, oxygen, hydrogen, nitrogen, sulfur, phosphorus, and a little iron. Water supplies building material and regulates the body's processes. It makes up the principal part of all the body fluids and secretion and helps make it possible for the body to regulate its own temperature.

Vitamins are found in raw and fresh vegetables, fruits, and grains, next to the outer coverings of grains and the peelings of fruits and vegetables. Vitamins are also found in the heart of grains and fruits.

Foods rich in carbohydrates: malt sugar, malt honey, ripe fruits, starchy vegetables, such as potatoes and cereals. These furnish energy and fuel.

Foods rich in proteins and carbohydrates: peas, beans, lentils, peanuts, oatmeal, and wheat furnish fuel and tissue building material.

Starchless vegetables: carrots, young beets, celery, cucumbers, tomatoes, soybean, squash, turnips, rutabagas, onions, okra, Brussels sprouts, and artichokes, furnish bulk.

Starchless and sugarless vegetables: lettuce, spinach, all greens, tomatoes, celery, radishes, beans (string), cabbage, cauliflower, eggplant, endive, and asparagus, furnish bulk.

Iron is found in spinach, dried peas, dried beans, whole wheat, prunes, watercress, celery cabbage, oats, lettuce, raisins, apples, English walnuts, lentils, and all greens.

Phosphorus is included in legumes, prunes, baked potatoes, nuts, whole cereals, cheese, soybean, and cottage cheese.

Calcium resides in whole cereals, cabbage, parsnips, citrus fruits, nuts, legumes, and soybean milk.

Magnesium can be found in cherries, apples, nuts, figs, raisins, turnips, prunes, legumes, spinach, natural brown rice, and whole cereals.

Potassium is in cherries, potatoes, parsnips, turnips, apples, plums, red cabbage, eggplants, cucumbers, and soybeans.

Sodium is in strawberry, apples, asparagus, spinach, and cauliflower.

Chlorine is found in spinach, cabbage, turnips, and cauliflower.

Sulfur is included in broccoli, cauliflower, cabbage, Brussels sprouts, kale, callaloo, spinach, asparagus, okra, lettuce, sweet corn, and eggplant.

Lime can be found in cabbage, cheese, all greens, legumes, and soybeans.

Fluorine is in cauliflower, cabbage, asparagus, potatoes, and spinach.

Selenium is in soybeans, tofu, nuts, seeds, barley, oats, cabbage, and spinach.

The foods highest in **iodine** include seaweed, prunes, lima beans, carrots, bananas, cucumber, sweet pepper, round tomato, cherry tomato, baked potato with peel, and navy beans.

Calcium builds bones and teeth. Whole cereals and fruits, especially citrus fruits, provide fluorine and silica, which are also needed for teeth and bones.

The primary functions of potassium in the body include regulating fluid balance and controlling the electrical activity of the heart and other muscles. Potassium supports blood pressure, cardiovascular health, bone strength, and muscle strength. Foods containing the highest amounts of potassium include, beet greens, white beans, soy beans, and lima beans. *Medicalnewstoday.com*

Sodium is necessary for muscle contraction, nerve conduction and water balance in the body. Potassium and Sodium are electrolytes needed for the body to function normally and help maintain fluid and blood volume in the body. However, a person can get high blood pressure by consuming too much sodium and not enough potassium.

"Salt: The Role of Potassium and Sodium in Your Diet." Centers for Disease Control and Prevention, June 29, 2018, www.cdc.gov/salt/potassium.htm.

The body uses sulfur for various important functions, including building and repairing DNA, as well as protecting your cells against damage. Including enough sulfur-rich foods in the diet is vital to health. Some foods rich in sulfur are: legumes; especially soybeans, black beans, kidney beans, split peas, and white beans, nuts and seeds; especially almonds, Brazil nuts, peanuts, walnuts, and pumpkin and sesame seeds, dried fruit; especially dried peaches, apricots, sultanas, and figs, certain vegetables; particularly asparagus, broccoli, Brussels sprouts, red cabbage, leeks, onion, radishes, turnip tops, and watercress, certain grains; especially pearl barley, oats, wheat, and flour made from these grains, condiments and spices. *Healthline.com*

The fundamental principle of true healing consists of a return to the natural habits of living. Our most common and serious disease are caused by wrong eating and drinking habits. This has been proven by numerous scientific experiments in recent years. Food is a substance which when absorbed by the blood stream will nourish, repair, and furnish life force and heat to the body. But if in its preparation and refining, the life-giving elements are taken away, will clog the functional activity of the body and will result in many disorders. Many diseases are nature's effort to free the system from poisons and congestions resulting from wrong eating and drinking. But when one assists nature to expel impurities and re-establish right conditions in the system, it is possible to overcome disease.

Since the first surrender to appetite, man has been growing more and more self-indulgent, until health is being sacrificed on the altar of appetite. *Christian Temperance and Bible Hygiene, pp 42, 43.* God gave the first parents the food He designed the human race to eat.

Vitamins for Older People

What vitamins should an elderly person take? This question is best answered by the family physician. Nutritional deficiencies are only too common in those who are older. A few vitamin pills will not necessarily solve the problem. One must be prepared to follow a sensible program of living. In the long run, a balanced diet is far more important than the addition of a few vitamin pills once or twice a day.

Most elderly people do not tolerate medicines as well as they did when they were younger. In many of these older people, the liver does not work so well. In life, the body depends upon the liver to change the chemicals of harmful drugs and render them harmless. In their later years, most people suddenly feel the urge to take more medicines. They are anxious to restore their lost energies. Many of them will swallow almost anything suggested on the television. This is hard on the liver. Many medicines that are commonly used today contain drugs there is no reason to load the system with. The common practice of loading the body with powerful chemicals, when something less potent would suffice is the norm of today. Before resorting to powerful drugs, why not consider some simpler less dangerous ways of relieving pain? Warm moist packs, a heating lamp, or fomentations will often relieve the pain. Cool wet dressing will usually bring comfort from severe itching and burning in the skin. Hydrotherapy is like magic of water, hot or cold, and is very beneficial in treating pain.

Part Eight:

Miracles in the Kitchen

(Recipes)

Hippocrates, the great Greek physician once said: "Let food be your medicine and medicine your food." It was good advice then and it is still good advice today, though few people take it to heart. Most doctors today prefer to prescribe expensive pills, painful shots, and high-tech tests to diagnose and treat what ails. However, cures can be found right in the kitchen cabinet.

Since the first born on planet earth, food has been the medicine and energy source. The animals have always known exactly which plants to eat when they're sick. All ancient civilizations from the Chinese to Native Americans have studied plants for their medicinal properties.

As civilization began to grow and flourish, plants remain the primary pharmacology. Hippocrates realized the value of herbal medicine early and prescribed it freely for a wide variety of illnesses. Respiratory disorders, for example, were treated with a combination of vinegar and cayenne pepper, which helped ease congestion and improved breathing. Galen, one of ancient Rome's most renowned physicians often recommended garlic for chest pain. In the middle ages, a heavy dose of mustard was the treatment of the day for coughs, asthma, and congestion.

Garlic

Garlic is a natural antibiotic for bacterial, viral, and fungus infections, and is an anti-cancer agent. It reduces high blood pressure and cholesterol levels. Use garlic for colds and flu. It aids asthma, colitic arthritis, chronic bronchitis, tonsillitis. Garlic contains vitamin A, B-Complex, C, and most minerals. Garlic, honey, and apple cider vinegar are three of the most effective natural remedies available and they're often stronger when used in combination.

Garlic is among the few herbs that have a universal usage and recognition. Its daily usage aids and supports the body in ways that no other herb does.

Fresh Honey

Fresh honey is another natural remedy with a rich historical heritage as a natural cure-all. It is a lot easier to take than garlic. The ancient Egyptians, who seemed to know as much about herbal medicine as they did about construction astounding structures, valued honey very highly. The Egyptians also recognized honey as an essential natural cure-all. In fact, honey is mentioned nearly five hundred times in nine hundred remedies discussed in Smith Papyrus, an Egyptian medical document. "**Edwin Smith papyrus,** (*c.* 1600 bc), ancient Egyptian medical treatise, believed to be a copy of a work dating from *c.* 3000 bc. Apparently intended as a textbook on surgery, it begins with clinical cases of head injuries and works systematically down the body, describing in detail examination, diagnosis, treatment, and prognosis in each case. *The Editors of Encyclopaedia Britannica. "Edwin Smith papyrus." Encyclopaedia Britannica, March 17, 2016, www.britannica.com/topic/Edwin-Smith-papyrus.*

The ancient Greeks and Romans also valued honey very highly. Greek Mythology is filled with references to honey and honeybees. Greek physicians also knew the value of honey as an important nutrient, and their writings are filled with references to honey as a powerful medicinal agent. Common uses for honey included a salve for burns, and scrapes; an antibiotic for cuts and other wounds. "Hippocrates himself used honey and vinegar for pain, honey and water for thirst, and honey mixed with water and other substances for fever." *Patterson, Susan. "How to Heal Your Body with Raw Honey." The Alternative Daily, www.thealternativedaily.com/how-to-heal-body-with-raw-honey/.*

During wartime, honey was rubbed into wounds to fight infection, an effective therapy also practiced by battle weary Germans in World War I. The Bible says "My son, eat thou honey, because it is good; and the honeycomb, which is sweet to thy taste:" *Proverbs 24:13* They used the sweet syrup in cooking, fed it to sacred animals, and often used it as a tribute to a higher authority, or to pay a debt.

Honey is one of the sweetest foods produced by nature and one of the best for the body. It is known that honey is made from a wide variety of flowering plants; some of the most common includes: Acaia, a pale-yellow honey, Alfalfa, a mild honey, Clover, common varieties, Orange Blossom, very mild and light colored, Tulip Poplar, a very dark honey. There are many uses for honey. It is especially handy as an ingredient in baked goods. It makes a good substitute for plain sugar. Honey is also packed with nutrients, including ascorbic acid, riboflavin, thiamine, and trace minerals. Because it has a higher level of fructose than cane sugar, it is less likely to affect blood glucose levels, which is good news for diabetics. But, diabetics should consult their doctors. Honey is a carbohydrate, an excellent source of quick energy. In fact, athletes worldwide often gulp a quick dose to improve performance on the field because of its rapidly absorbed into the bloodstream. When a calcium supplement is taken with honey, the glucose in the honey increases the body's uptake of the mineral by as much as twenty-five percent. Honey also has a major role to play as a carrier of foods containing relatively high levels of vitamins and minerals, and has been shown to help the body absorb minerals such as calcium. *Tan, Ruth. "5 Key Health Benefits of Honey." Benefits of Honey, www.benefits-of-honey.com/health-benefits-of-honey.html.*

Pasta Salad

2 medium green bell peppers diced
1 medium red bell pepper diced
1 medium yellow onion diced
1 large cucumber diced
1 medium red onion diced
2 medium tomatoes cut in chunks
1 cup veggie cheese
½ cup Italian dressing
1 teaspoon olive oil
Salt to taste
Cayenne pepper to taste
1 - 8-ounce box of spaghetti

Cook spaghetti adding the 1 teaspoon olive oil to water to prevent sticking. Drain and strain in cool water. Add all ingredients except the cheese and dressing and mix thoroughly. Add dressing and cheese and serve.

Artichoke Mushroom Salad

14 ounce can artichoke hearts
½ pound fresh mushrooms or 8 ounce can
2 cloves crushed garlic
1 teaspoon of thyme
1 tablespoon of veggie mayonnaise

Combine all ingredients and marinate in veggie mayonnaise in the refrigerator for one half hour. Serve over bed of lettuce.

Raw Broccoli Salad

1 head of broccoli
½ cup chopped olives
½ cup onion chopped
½ cup carrots shredded
1 cup artichoke half
½ cup veggie mayonnaise
Salt and pepper to taste

Mix well and let set refrigerated for one half hour. Serve.

Sour Kraut Salad

2 cups or 16 ounces of kraut drained
1 cup onion chopped
1 cup green bell pepper chopped
1 cup celery chopped
1 cup pimentos

Dressing

½ cup lemon juice
2 tablespoons water
1 cup olive oil
1 ½ cup raw sugar

Bring to boil all liquid ingredients. Stir in raw sugar and stir until dissolved. Put all other ingredients into one bowl and pour dressing over vegetables while hot. Cool in refrigerator for 24 hours. Serve cold.

Melon Salad

½ of medium watermelon chunked
1 honey dew melon
1 cantaloupe chunked
3 cups sliced cherries
1 pineapple chunked
½ pound black grapes

Mix all together.

A Diet Salad

¼ cabbage grated fine
1 large apple grated
¼ fresh pineapple grated fine
10 ounce black and red grapes sliced

Mix all together.

Sauce for Diet Salad

2 ounces pineapple juice
3 pitted dates

Blend until smooth and pour over salad.

Fruit Platter

Cut 3 oranges into wedges with rinds still on
Cut 2 grapefruits into wedges with rinds still on
1 cup of fresh sliced strawberries or grapes

Wash fruit thoroughly before cutting. Arrange alternately on a platter in a circle, placing the strawberries or grapes in the center of the circle; this makes an attractive center piece.

Banana Ice Cream

Peel 6 - 8 bananas

Place in a freezer storage bag and leave in freezer until thoroughly frozen. Place frozen bananas in blender with a small amount of fruit juice. Blend until consistency of ice cream. Top with granola or chopped walnuts.

You may use any combination of frozen fruit to make ice cream.

Simple Apple Salad

3 apples cored and diced
½ cup raisins
½ cup shredded coconut
½ cup sunflower seeds

Mix all ingredients together in a bowl. Add pineapple or lemon juice to prevent discoloration.

Fruit Soup

2 ½ cups pineapple juice
2 ½ tablespoons Minute Tapioca
½ cup raisins
1 apple diced with peel still on
2 - 16 ounce can of peach halves
2 bananas sliced
½ cup strawberries or raspberries

Cook tapioca in pineapple juice until it thickens. Mix tapioca in a bowl with raisins, peaches, and apples. Add banana slices over top when ready to serve.

Rice and Cashew Casserole

2 cups cooked rice
1 cup chopped celery
½ chopped onion
1/3 cup soy milk
½ cup cashews
1 can mushroom soup
1 - 4 ounce can mushroom
½ cup mayonnaise

Mix all ingredients together. Place in oiled casserole dish. Sprinkle with paprika. Bake at 350 for 45 minutes.

Baked Stuffing

9 cups fluffy bread crumbs
2 teaspoons sage
1 onion minced
1 cup chopped celery
¼ to ½ cup vegetable margarine
1 cup cold water
3 tablespoons agar agar or egg substitute
Salt to taste

Mix bread crumbs with sage, salt, and chopped celery. Melt margarine and add minced onion. Cook on stove until limp but not brown. Remove from heat. Add cold water and agave together then mix in crumbs and mix well. Add water to make moist but not wet. Spread in well-oiled flat pan and bake at 350 degrees for thirty minutes.

Hummus Sandwich Spread

4 cups cooked garbanzos drained/blend save juice
2 - 4 cloves garlic minced
1 cup sesame seeds
2 - 3 tablespoons soy sauce
1 1/2 teaspoons onion powder
2 teaspoons cumin powder

Place sesame seeds in blender and grind into meal. Add together all ingredients except garbanzos. Add bean liquid to make a thick paste. Add paste to beans and mix together. Salt to taste. You may add finely chopped onions, parsley, celery and olives. Spread on whole grain bread and serve with lettuce, tomatoes and sprouts.

Chili

4 cups cooked kidney beans
4 cups cooked pinto beans
1 cup celery
1 cup onions
1 medium green pepper
2 cloves garlic
1 ½ teaspoons cumin
1 tablespoon sweet basil chopped
1 teaspoon onion powder
2 tablespoons honey
1 ½ teaspoons oregano
1 ½ quart tomatoes
Salt to taste

Sauté onion, celery, pepper, and garlic then add seasonings. Put in pot with the beans and tomatoes and simmer until all ingredients are well blended. Add tomato paste if a thicker consistency is desired.

Big Pot of Veggie Chili

5 cups cooked pinto beans
5 cups cooked black bens
2 - 28-ounce cans diced tomatoes
1 - 12 ounce can tomato paste
10 cups water
1/3 cup olive oil
1 green bell pepper chopped
1 yellow bell pepper chopped
1 red bell pepper chopped
2 large jalapeno peppers (remove seeds if less heat is required)
3 medium onions
6 clove garlic
4 tablespoons chili powder
2 tablespoons cumin
1 teaspoon onion powder
1 teaspoon garlic powder
1 bunch of cilantro finely chopped

Combine first 5 ingredients in large pot. Sauté the peppers and onions in a large skillet until they are slightly translucent before adding the garlic. When garlic is slightly brown add all, including the oil, to the bean mixture. Stir in all seasonings including chopped cilantro. Cover and simmer over medium heat for 45 minutes. Check frequently for consistency. Add water if needed. Taste and adjust seasonings as your taste demands.

Tofu Burgers

¼ cup chopped onions
¼ cup chopped celery
1 cup cooked brown rice
1 cup mashed tofu
1 cup bean sprouts
½ cup whole wheat bread crumbs
1 ½ teaspoon soy sauce

Slightly chop bean sprouts. Sauté onion and celery and combine with other ingredients. Press into patties and place on oiled baking sheet. Bake in oven at 350 for 20 minutes until brown. Makes 4 servings.

Walnut Roast

2 cups soy milk
4 cups crushed corn flakes
1 onion chopped
½ teaspoon sage
¾ cup ground walnuts
1 tablespoon olive oil

Simmer onion in oil and add a little water. Mix all ingredients together. Put olive oil in loaf pan then add all ingredients. Bake at 350 for one hour.

Oat Burgers

4 ½ cups water
½ cup soy sauce
4 ½ cup rolled oats
1/3 cup oil
1 diced onion
1 teaspoon garlic powder
¼ cup Brewer's yeast
¼ cup sesame seeds
¾ cup chopped nuts

Bring water and soy sauce to boil. Add rolled oats and cook for five minutes. Sit the oats aside to cool. Sauté other ingredients and add to cooled oats. Form patties and bake at 350 for 30 to 45 minutes. Turn every 15 minutes. [Yeast flakes may be used instead of Brewer's Yeast.) Makes 20 patties.

Pasta Sauce

1 cup onion chopped
1 cup mushrooms chopped
½ cup carrots finely chopped
6 cups tomato sauce
5 cloves garlic minced
2 tablespoons basil
1 tablespoon rosemary
½ teaspoon thyme
½ teaspoon marjoram
½ teaspoon dry mustard

In large pan cook onions, mushrooms, and carrots until tender. Add remaining ingredients. Cook one hour stirring occasionally. Yield 5 cups. Cook one day before using to allow flavors to blend well.

Baked Noodles with Yogurt

¾ cup plain vegan Greek yogurt
½ cup green onions sliced
3 cups cooked whole wheat elbow pasta
1 cup onions chopped
1 cup sliced mushrooms
2 tablespoons water
½ teaspoon garlic minced
½ teaspoon oregano
½ teaspoon dried basil
1 ¼ cup pasta sauce (recipe in book)
1 ½ teaspoon honey
5 ounces veggie cheese shredded

Preheat oven at 350. In medium bowl combine yogurt, green onion and cooked pasta. Mix well and set aside. In medium sauce pan, simmer onion and mushrooms in 2 tablespoons water until tender. Add garlic, oregano, basil, pasta sauce and honey. Mix well. Put pasta mixture in 10x6x2 inch glass casserole dish. Top with sauce mixture and sprinkle with cheese. Bake at 350 for 20 minutes. Yield 8 servings.

Veggie Rice Casserole

2 cups cooked brown rice
1 cup grated veggie cheese
½ chopped onion
1 cup cauliflower flowerets
1 cup chopped broccoli
½ cup sliced celery
½ cup carrots sliced
½ cup zucchini sliced
2 cups pasta sauce (recipe in book)
1 clove garlic minced
2 teaspoons dried basil

Preheat to 350. Combine rice and half of cheese, mix well. Place in well-oiled 10/6/2 inch baking dish. Meanwhile, steam vegetables 5 to 7 minutes until tender and crisp then spoon vegetables over rice cheese mixture. Combine pasta sauce, garlic, and basil. Pour over vegetables and top with remaining cheese. Bake for 30 minutes. Yield 8 servings.

Stuffed Green Peppers

3 cups raw brown rice
4 green peppers
1 cup water
1 teaspoon safflower oil
½ cup onion chopped
½ cup celery chopped
½ cup mushrooms chopped
½ vegetable seasoning
½ teaspoon oregano
1/3 cup parsley chopped
3 cups pasta sauce (recipe in book)
4 ounces veggie cheese shredded
1 tablespoon wheat germ

Cook rice according to directions. Cut peppers in half lengthwise. Remove seeds and blanch in water until tender. Rinse peppers and set aside. Preheat oven to 375. Heat oil in a medium skillet and sauté onions, celery, mushrooms, seasonings, and parsley. Add to rice with one cup of tomato sauce and cheese and mix well. Stuff peppers with mixture and top with remaining tomato sauce. Sprinkle wheat germ and cheese. Bake at 375 for 35 minutes. Spoon sauce over each pepper and serve. Yield 4 servings.

Vegetable Stew

1 ½ tablespoons olive oil
1 medium onion sliced
2 cloves garlic minced
1 ½ pound diced eggplant
2 tablespoons fresh bay leaves chopped
1 teaspoon lemon peel grated
1 cup plain vegan Greek yogurt
1 teaspoon mustard
1 teaspoon horseradish
½ teaspoon honey
3 medium tomatoes peeled and chopped

Put olive oil in a large sauce pan and heat over medium high heat. Sauté onion and garlic until tender. Add eggplant, zucchini, parsley, basil and lemon peel and reduce heat. Let simmer for 20 minutes until eggplant is tender. Combine yogurt, mustard, horseradish, and honey in a small bowl. Cover and chill. Add tomatoes to the stew and continue cooking for 5 more minutes. Serve hot topped with dollop of yogurt dressing. Yield 6 servings.

Quick Lentil Casserole

2 cups cooked brown rice
1 - 10-ounce package frozen corn drained
1 - 15 ounce can of Con Health Valley Chili with Lentils
4-ounce firm tofu drained
¼ cup Daiya cheese shredded

Preheat oven 350. Mix rice, corn, chili and tofu in a medium bowl. Spoon mixture into an oiled casserole dish. Sprinkle with cheese. Bake for 15 minutes or until warmed through. Yield 6 servings.

Yummy Peanut Butter Bars

1 cup of coconut sugar packed
½ cup peanut butter
2 teaspoons vegan butter
¼ cup egg substitute
½ cup coconut milk
1 teaspoon vanilla extract
1 cup rolled oats
½ cup unbleached flour
1 teaspoon aluminum-free baking powder
½ teaspoon salt
1 cup dried plums

Preheat oven at 350. In mixer bowl beat together sugar, peanut butter, and margarine at medium speed until creamy. Add milk, egg substitute, and vanilla beat well combine oats, flour, baking powder and salt. Add peanut butter mixture. Mix until blended. Stir in dried plums. Press evenly into well-greased pan and bake 24 to 27 minutes or until golden brown. Yield 32 servings.

Low-Fat Fruit Smoothie

1 cup papayas chopped
1 cup mango chopped
½ cup water or apple juice
½ cup ice cubes
1 teaspoon vanilla extract
1 ½ coconut milk

Place all ingredients in a blender and blend until smooth. Yields 4 servings.

Carrot Soufflé

7 cups chopped carrots
2/3 cup raw sugar
½ cup soy cream
3 tablespoons unbleached flour
2 tablespoons vegan butter melted
1 teaspoon vanilla extract
¼ teaspoon salt
3 tablespoons agave
1 teaspoon raw sugar

Cook carrots in boiling water for 15 minutes until very tender. Drain and place carrots in food processor and blend until smooth. Add raw sugar, soy cream, flour, vegetable butter, vanilla extract, and salt. Blend together agave and brown sugar. Place mixture of agave and raw sugar in bottom of greased baking dish. Spoon in carrot mixture onto of the mixture. Bake at 350 for 40 minutes or until puffed and set.

Index

P

R

S

T

U

V

W

Made in the USA
Monee, IL
04 November 2026

67382369R00095